Key Notes

for

Anesthesia Oral Board

Z. Guan, M.D.

Assistant Professor
Department of Anesthesia & Perioperative Care
UCSF
San Francisco, California

Printed in the United States of America
ISBN-13: 978-1-4486-2123-1
ISBN-10: 1-4486-2123-2

Every effort has been exerted to assure the completeness and accuracy of the information contained within this book. However, in view of ongoing research, and the constant flow of information relating to the practice of medicine, the reader is urged to exert professional responsibility when applying this information in a particular situation or clinical circumstance. The author or the publisher are not responsible for errors or omissions or for any negative consequences from the application of the information contained within this book. Medicine is an ever changing field and no warranty is expressed or implied with respect to the currency, completeness, or the accuracy of the contents of this publication.

Table of Contents

Preface – Advices for Anesthesia Oral Board

1. Anesthesia oral board is to test your judgment, adaption, clarity, and application in clinical anesthesia. The knowledge base for oral board is very different from that tested by written board. In written board you can have rather vague knowledge to be able to pick up the right answers, whereas in oral board you have to have well organized and clear-cut knowledge to be able to speak it out.

2. Usually the answers in oral board need to be short and right to the point, simply because a lot of questions will be asked in a short period of time. In the ABA sample examination, nearly 170 questions are asked in 70 minutes. That is less than 25 seconds a question on average, including the time the questions are asked!

3. As a result, the knowledge base for oral board has to be concise and precise. To fulfill this goal, the Key Notes contains only key facts of all major clinical anesthesia scenarios, and it is organized in clinically related categories or systems in such ways that it is easy to remember and easy to speak out. It also contains ASA guidelines and the most important results from the recent major studies. In addition to oral board preparation, the Key Notes can also be used as a quick clinical reference book for daily anesthesia practice.

4. Because the oral board is testing your ability to express your opinions, it would be better to prepare for it by reading out loud and speaking up load this Key Notes as often as you can until you can totally memorize it.

5. Although all aspects of clinical anesthesia are important for oral board, you should pay particular attention to airway related topics, because they are the topics of the highest yield.

6. You should have sufficient mock oral tests to get familiar with the pace and the format, and to get used to speaking in front of other people. However, you will benefit the most from these mock tests only after you have memorized the Key Notes.

7. In addition to the Key Notes, consider review the materials you used for your written board to cover the low yield topics. Because you are already quite familiar with those materials, it will be more efficient to go through them than reading a new big oral board review book. It seems unlikely that the oral board will ask you any question that is not even covered by the written board.

8. In the exam, you will have two 35-minute sessions, tested by two examiners in each session. The first session has a long stem case that has intraoperative (10 minutes), postoperative (15 minutes), and additional topic questions (10 min). The second session has a short stem case that has preoperative (10 minutes), intraoperative (15 minutes), and additional topic questions (10 minutes). You will have about 10 minutes to prepare for each case. During this time, you should at least think thoroughly about the induction and airway issues. It is almost guaranteed that it will be tested in almost every single case.

9. In general, do not ask examiners questions about the case. It is just a waste of your precious time because they simply do not know the answer. The information you have about the case is all they have. If you definitely need some critical information, just assume it by saying "Assuming", such as "Assuming blood pressure is OK, ..." or "Assuming airway is good, ..."
10. In general, do not argue with the examiners.
11. There are two most common types of questions in oral board: "What do you think?" questions and "What do you do?" questions.
12. "What do you think?" questions ask you about the differentials. Your first answer should always be the most like differential in this case at this point. If your first shot hits the target (the answer the examiners are looking for), the examination will quickly move on to next question.
13. You should go to your extensive differential lists only after you miss the target with your first shot. Even in this situation you should organize your differentials in categories such as systems. This will not only help you to memorize these differentials, more importantly it will also show the examiners that you have clear clinical thinking.
14. To answer "What do you do?" questions, you should always organize your thoughts in the following five steps: confirm, check vital sign, immediate rescue management, differential, and specific treatment according to the differential.
15. If you don't know the answer of a question, simply say "I don't know" so that the examiners can quickly move on to next question that you might get credit from.
16. Do not panic if you miss a few questions in your exam. Nearly everyone misses at least one question.
17. If you think you might fail the first part of the exam, do not give up on your second part. You will be amazed to find out how many examinees actually pass the exam when they think they might have failed it.
18. The passing rate is ~ 80% for all first takers and ~ 55% for all repeaters.

Chapter 1 Essential Topics

Monitors

1. ASA standard monitors (2003):
   a. BP cuff
   b. EKG
   c. Pulse oximeter (SpO_2 90% is ~ PaO_2 65 mmHg)
   d. T
   e. Capnography
   f. Oxygen analyzer
   *Twitch monitor (not an ASA standard monitor)
2. Invasive monitor
   a. A-line:
      - Indication
        - Any patient with severe cardiovascular disease
        - Any bloody surgery
        - Real time BP monitor
        - ABG and other lab sampling
   b. Central line:
      - Indication
        - Preload monitor (CVP > 12 mmHg indicates overload)
          a. Measure at end of expiration between a & c waves
        - Medication route
   c. PA catheter
      - Indication
        - Wedge pressure (nl < 15 mmHg, > 18 mmHg indicates significant LV malfunction; measure at end of expiration)
        - CO (nl 4-6 L/min; index nl 3-4 $L/min/m^2$)
        - Pulm HTN (nl systolic < 30 mmHg)
        - SvO_2 (nl 70%)
          a. best way to access CO in absence of hypoxia and severe anemia
        - Pacing
   d. Foley
3. Specific monitor
   a. EEG, SSEP, MEP
   b. ICP
   c. Precordial Doppler
   d. BIS
   e. TEE
   f. Fetal monitor

Airway Management (ASA 2003 Guideline)

History
1. h/o difficult airway
2. OSA
3. Hoarseness
4. Dysphonia
5. Dysphagia
Patient might be difficult in mask vent

Pre-op airway physical examination
1. Mouth
   a. Mouth opening
   b. Upper incisors
   c. Interincisor distance
   d. Tongue
   e. Mallampati (uvula & palate)
2. Neck
   a. Thyromental distance
   b. ROM
   c. Length of neck
   d. Thickness of neck

Five major eval:
1. Difficulty in mask ventilation
2. Difficulty in intubation
3. Difficulty in patient cooperation
4. Risk of aspiration
5. Difficulty in tracheostomy

Four major questions:
1. RSI? Sux vs. rocuronium?
2. Awake FOI?
3. Spontaneous breathing (Inhalation vs. ketamine)?
4. Invasive technique (tracheostomy vs. cricothyrotomy)?

Techniques for difficult ventilation
1. Chin lift, jaw thrust
2. Oral and/or nasal airway
3. LMA
4. Call for help /two-person mask ventilation
5. Cricothyrotomy with transtracheal jet ventilation
6. Tracheostomy

Techniques for Difficult Intubation
1. Different blade
2. FOI
3. Intubate through LMA (fast-track LMA, FOI through LMA)

4. Retrograde
5. Tracheostomy
6. Cancel case

Intraop Aspiration

NPO (ASA 1999 Guideline, all age)
1. Clear liquids – 2 h
2. Breast milk – 4 h
3. Infant formula – 6 h
4. Non-human milk – 6 h
5. Light meal – 6 h
   * Big fatty meal – 8h
   * Pain and narcotics delays gastric emptying

Prevention
1. NPO
2. Medical prophylaxis
   a. Bicitra 30 ml PO
   b. Reglan 10 mg iv
   c. Zantac 50 mg iv
3. Gastric tube
4. RSI with cricoid pressure vs. awake FOI

What do you do for intra-op aspiration?
1. T-bug and head to the side
2. Suction
3. RSI with cricoid pressure
4. Vent with 100% $\pm$ PEEP
5. Bronchoscopy
6. NGT
7. ABG, CXR
8. No antibiotic, steroid, or irrigation

Hypoxia (Low SpO_2)

What do you think (differential)?
I think the most likely the cause in this case is ___, other differential includes:
1. Artifacts
   a. Sensor misplacement
   b. Low temperature
   c. Hypotension
   d. Methylene blue
2. Low FiO_2
3. Hypoventilation

    a. Airway obstruction: ETT kinked, Mucous plug
    b. Ventilator disconnection or failure
    c. ↓ Respiratory drive: depression (i.e. drugs) or failure (i.e. paralysis) in pt with spontaneous breathing
4. Shunt & V/Q mismatch (nl 0.8)
    a. One lung vent /ETT too deep (main stem intubation)
    b. PTX
    c. Lung problems: pulmonary edema, atelectasis, pneumonia
    d. Cardiac right-to-left shunt
5. Hb
    a. Methemoglobinemia

What do you do? (Confirm, Check, Rescue, Differential, Treatment)
1. Confirm: check pulse oximeter sensor
2. Check:
    a. ASA standard monitor
    b. Vt, airway pressure, breath sound bilateral
3. Rescue:
    a. ↑ FiO_2
    b. Add PEEP
    c. Hand vent with 100% O_2 if necessary
4. Differential:
5. Specific Treatment: ETT adjust, ETT suction, scope, albuterol ... (depends on etiology)

Hypercarbia

What do you think (differential)?
I think the most likely the cause in this case is ___, other differential includes:
1. Low minutes ventilation
    a. Inadequate vent setting
    b. Airway obstruction
    c. Decreased compliance
    d. Decrease resp. drive (spontaneous breathing)
    e. Muscle weakness (spontaneous breathing)
2. Increased CO_2 production
    a. MH
    b. Neuroleptic malignant syndrome
    c. Burn
    d. Shiver
    e. Fever
    f. Seizure
3. Rebreathing
    a. Exhausted soda lime
    b. Incompetent inspiratory or expiratory check valve
4. Surgery related
    a. Tourniquet or aortic cross-clamp release

      b. CO_2 absorption (pneumoperitoneum for laparoscopic procedures)

What do you do? (Confirm, Check, Rescue, Differential, Treatment)
1. Confirm
2. Check
    a. ASA standard monitor
    b. Vt, airway pressure, breath sound bilateral
3. Rescue: ↑ Vm, hand vent if necessary
4. Differential
5. Specific treatment

Increase Airway Pressure

What do you think (differential)?
I think the most likely the cause in this case is ___, other differential includes:
1. Machine
    a. Expiratory valve prolapse
2. ETT
    a. Kinked ETT
    b. Deep intubation
    c. Mucous plug
    d. Herniated cuff
3. Bronchospasm
    a. Asthma
    b. COPD
    c. Aspiration
    d. Allergic reaction
4. Respiratory
    a. Pulmonary edema
    b. PTX /PE
    c. Rigid chest wall from narcotics
5. Breathing against vent

What do you do?
1. Confirm: hand vent with 100% O_2
2. Check
    a. ASA standard monitor
    b. Vt, breath sound bilateral
3. Rescue:
    a. ↑ Depth of anesthesia
    b. ↑ FiO_2
    c. Hand vent with 100% O_2
4. Differential
5. Specific treatment

Wheezing

What do you think (differential)?

I think the most likely the cause in this case is ___, other differential includes:

1. Lower airway /ETT
    a. ETT
        - Kinked ETT
        - Bronchial intubation
    b. Bronchial
        - Bronchospasm
        - Aspiration
        - Mucous plug
        - Anaphylactic reaction
        - Foreign body
    c. Lung
        - Pneumonia
        - Pulmonary edema
        - PTX
        - PE
2. Upper airway
    a. Supraglottic
        - Big tongue
        - Foreign body
        - Polyps
    b. Glottic
        - Laryngospasm
        - Laryngeal edema
        - Vocal cord paralysis

What do you do? (Confirm, Check, Rescue, Differential, Treatment)

1. Confirm: Bilateral wheezing? Chest rise?
2. Check
    a. ASA standard monitor
    b. Vt, airway pressure, breath sound bilateral
3. Rescue
    a. Deepen anesthesia
    b. ↑ FiO_2
    c. Add PEEP
    d. Albuterol
    e. Hand vent with 100% O_2
    f. Epinephrine or ephedrine iv
    g. Steroid
4. Differential
5. Specific treatment

Hypotension

What do you think (differential)?
I think the most likely the cause in this case is ___, other differential includes:
1. Anesthesia related
   a. Anesthetic overdose
   b. Anti-hypertensive medication overdose
2. Surgery related
   a. Hypovolemia
   b. Compression of IVC, heart, aorta cross-clamp
   c. Cross-clamp relief
3. Cardiac
   a. Pre-load
      - Hypovolemia
      - PE
      - PTX
      - Tamponade
      - IVC/SVC compression
   b. Pump
      - CHF
      - MI
      - Dysrhythmia
      - Valvular dysfunction
   c. After-load
      - Shock: anaphylactic, septic, neurogenic (cord injury)
4. Pulmonary
   a. Hypoxia
   b. Hypercarbia
5. Other (think about ASA monitors and labs you send)
   a. Hypothermia
   b. Hyper/hypokalemia
   c. Hypoglycemia
   d. Acidosis

What do you do? (Confirm, Check, Rescue, Differential, Treatment)
1. Confirm: check pulse, recycle BP cuff, flush AL, check transducer location
2. Check:
   a. ASA standard monitor
   b. Vt, airway pressure, breath sound bilateral
3. Rescue
   a. CPR if necessary
   b. Reduce anesthesia
   c. Medication: ephedrine, phenylephrine …
   d. IV fluid
4. Differential
5. Specific treatment

Pulseless Arrest

What do you do? (ACLS 2005)
1. CPR
2. Check ASA standard monitor: ECG (rhythm, HR), BP, SpO_2, T, O_2, CO_2; & breath sound bilateral
    a. VF/VT (Shockable)
        - Give 1st shock
            • Biphase 120-200 J
            • Monophase 360 J
        - Resume CPR immediately for 2 min
        - Check pulse
        - Lab if have time: ABG, CBC, Chem7
        - Check rhythm
        - Give 2nd shock if VF/VT persists
            • Biphase 200 J
            • Monophase 360 J
        - Resume CPR immediately for 2 min
        - *Epinephrine* 1 mg IV q3-5 min prn
        - Check pulse
        - Check rhythm
        - Give 3rd shock if VT/VF persists
        - Resume CPR immediately for 2 min
        - *Lidocaine* 1 mg/kg IV, then 0.5 mg/kg, max 3 mg/kg
            • (or *Amiodarone* 300 mg IV followed by 150 mg)
        - *Magnesium* 2g IV for torsades de pointes
        - Check pulse
        - Check rhythm
    b. Asystole/PEA (Not shockable)
        - CPR 2 min
        - Lab: ABG, CBC, Chem 7
        - *Epinephrine* 1 mg IV q3-5 min prn
        - Atropine 1 mg IV q3-5 min (Max X 3) if asystole or slow rate PEA
        - Check pulse
        - Check rhythm
        - Cont. CPR if asystole/PEA persists
3. Concerns about CPR
    a. 100 pushes/min
    b. 2 min mark
        - CPR 5 cycles
        - Check rhythm q2 min
        - Rotate compressors q2 min
    c. Avoid hyperventilation

What do you think (differential)? Same differential as for hypotension.

10

Hypertension

What do you think (differential)?
I think the most likely the cause in this case is ___, other differential includes:
1. Anesthesia related
    a. Inadequate anesthesia
    b. Inadequate pain control
    c. Vasopressor overdose
2. Surgery related
    a. Tourniquet
    b. Aortic cross-clamp
    c. Pheochromocytoma dissection
3. Cardiac
    a. Baseline HTN
    b. Volume overload
4. Pulm
    a. Hypoxia
    b. Hypercarbia
5. Neuro
    a. Increased ICP
    b. Carotid sinus resection bil.
6. Endo
    a. Pheochromocytoma
    b. Carcinoid
    c. Thyroid storm
7. Drug effect
    a. Drug withdrawal
    b. Cocaine
    c. MAOI with demerol
    d. Pheochromocytoma + droperidol

What do you do?
1. Confirm: recycle BP cuff, check AL transducer location
2. Check
    a. ASA standard monitors
    b. Vt, airway pressure, breath sound bilateral
3. Rescue
    a. Increase anesthesia
    b. Better pain control
    c. Labetalol if HR is OK
    d. Nitroglycerine
    e. Nitroprusside
4. Differential
5. Specific treatment

Tachycardia

What do you think (differential)?
I think the most likely the cause in this case is ___, other differential includes:

1. Anesthesia related
    a. Inadequate anesthesia
    b. Inadequate pain control
    c. Intra-op medication: anticholinergics, pancuronium, histamine release
    d. Bladder distension
2. Surgery related
    a. Bleeding
    b. Decrease venous return: IVC compression
    c. Cross-clamp relief
3. Cardiovascular
    a. Pre-load
        -   Hypovolemia
        -   PE
        -   PTX
        -   Tamponade
    b. Pump
        -   Dysrhythmia: SVT, A-fib, A flut, VT…
        -   MI
        -   Pacer malfunction
    c. After-load
        -   Hypotension
4. Pulm
    a. Hypoxia
    b. Hypercarbia
5. Drug effect
    a. Drug withdrawal: clonidine, ETOH
    b. MAOI + demerol
    c. Pheochromocytoma + droperidol
6. Endo
    a. MH
    b. Neuroleptic Malignant Syndrome
    c. Thyroid storm
    d. Carcinoid
    e. Pheochromocytoma
    f. Fever
    g. Electrolyte problems

What do you do?
1. Confirm: check ECG, pulse
2. Check
    a. ASA standard monitor
    b. Vt, airway pressure, breath sound bilateral
3. Rescue

      a. CPR if no pulse

      b. Cardioversion

         - Afib: synchronized 50-100 J

         - Supraventricular tachy: synchronized 25-50 J

      c. Defibrilate if VT

      d. Adenosine for supraventricular tachycardia

      e. Temporally control with β blocker (esmolol) if BP is OK

4. Differential

      a. Labs: ABG, CBC, Chem7

5. Specific treatment

Dysrhythmia

What do you think (differential)?

I think the most likely the cause in this case is ___, other differential includes:

1. Anesthesia related
    a. Inadequate pain control
    b. Intra-op medication
2. Cardiac
    a. MI/ischemia
    b. Baseline conduction abnormalities
    c. Myocarditis
    d. HTN/hypotension
    e. Valvular disease
3. Pulmonary
    a. Hypoxia
    b. Hypercarbia
4. Electrolyte: K^+, Ca^{++}, Mg^{++}
5. Endo
    a. Hyperthyroidism
    b. Pheochromocytoma

What do you do?

1. Confirm: ECG, pulse
2. Check
    a. ASA standard monitor
    b. Vt, airway pressure, breath sound bilateral
3. Rescue
    a. CPR if unstable
    b. Lidocaine for PVC > 6/min
        - 1 mg/kg bolus
        - Another 0.5 mg/kg
        - Infusion 1 mg/min
4. Differential
    a. Labs: ABG, CBC, Electrolytes
    b. 12 lead ECG, CXR

5. Specific treatment

Bradycardia

What do you think (differential)?

I think the most likely the cause in this case is ___, other differential includes:

1. Anesthesia related
   a. Succinylcholine
   b. β blocker
   c. Neostigmine
   d. High spinal or spinal shock
   e. Opiates
   f. Hypothermia
2. Surgery related (vagal reflex)
   a. Carotid sinus stimulation
   b. Visceral traction
   c. Bladder distension
3. Cardiac
   a. Dysrhythmia: AVB, SSS
   b. MI
   c. Pacer malfunction
4. Pulmonary
   a. Hypoxia
   b. Hypercarbia
5. Neuro
   a. Increased ICP

What do you do?

1. Confirm: check pulse
2. Check
   a. ASA standard monitor
   b. Vt, airway pressure, breath sound bilateral
3. Rescue
   a. Drug: Ephedrine, glycopyrrolate, atropine
   b. Pacemaker
4. Differential
5. Specific treatment

Oliguria (< 0.5 ml/kg/hr)

What do you think (differential)?

I think the most likely the cause in this case is ___, other differential includes:

1. Pre-renal
   a. Hypovolemia
   b. Hypotension

      c. Renal artery or vein thrombosis /compression
2. Renal
      a. ATN
          - Myoglobinuria, hemoglobinuria
          - Contrast
          - Gentamicin (aminoglycosides)
      b. Intrinsic disease
          - CRF (HTN, DM)
3. Post-renal
      a. Foley obstruction or misplacement
      b. Urethral or ureteral obstruction

What do you do?
1. Confirm
2. Check
      a. ASA standard monitor
      b. Vt, airway pressure, breath sound bilateral
3. Rescue
      a. Check Foley
      b. Check volume status
      c. Fluid challenge of 250-500 ml
      d. Mannitol (lasix would not help to reserve renal function) ~ *lasix is OK*
      e. Fenoldopam
4. Differential
      a. BUN/Cr ratio: > 20 indicates prerenal
      b. FENa (Fraction excretion of sodium): < 1% indicates prerenal, > 3% renal
      c. Urine sodium: < 10 mEq/L indicated prerenal, > 40 indicates mEq/L renal
      d. Urine osmolarity and gravity
5. Specific treatment

Bleeding /Oozing

What do you think (differential)?
I think the most likely the cause in this case is ___, other differential includes:
1. Surgical bleeding
2. Platelet problem
      a. Bleeding time
      b. plt count
3. Factor problem
      a. PT/INR: Extrinsic (factor VII)
      b. PTT/**ACT** (heparin): Intrinsic (Factor VIII(**A**))
4. Heparin/coumadin
5. DIC
6. Transfusion hemolytic reaction
7. Hypothermia

Extubation Criteria

1. No risk of upper airway obstruction
   - Leak test ~ 20 cmH$_2$O
2. Vital signs stable
3. No repeat surgery in near future
4. Mental status: awake
5. Adequate strength
   a. Sustained tetanus for 5 s
   b. Equal double bursts
   c. Head lift for 5 s
   d. Equal TOF is not sufficient
6. Sufficient respiratory effort (ICU pt)
   a. Oxygenation: PaO$_2$ > 70 on FiO$_2$ 40%
   b. Ventilation: PaCO$_2$ < 55
   c. MIF more than -20 cmH$_2$O

Laryngeal Spasm

1. General
   a. Superior laryngeal nerve stimulation
   b. More common in pedi pts (1 in 50)
   c. Recent URI or 2nd hand smoking increases risk
2. Prevention
   a. Extubate either awake (opening eyes) or deep (spontaneous breathe without coughing or swallowing)
   b. Post-op lateral position in PACU (pedi pt)
3. Treatment
   a. Positive pressure ventilation
   b. Jaw thrust
   c. Small dose succinylcholine (0.5 mg/kg) iv
   d. Rocuronium (0.4 mg/kg) iv if sux in contraindicated
   e. Sux i.m. if no IV (10 times as iv, 5 mg/kg)
   f. Lidocaine iv (1 mg/kg) alternatively

Post-intubation Croup

1. Confirm: Chart review, assess pt, physical exam
2. Check: ASA standard monitor
3. Rescue
   a. 100% O$_2$ mask if necessary
   b. Intubate if necessary
   c. Racemic epinephrine nebulizer
   d. Decadron iv

4. Physiology
    a. Caused by glottis or trachea edema
    b. Appear within 3 h after extubation
    c. Associated with difficult intubation and large ETT

Prolonged Postop Apnea

What do you think (differential)?
I think the most likely the cause in this case is ___, other differential includes:
1. Airway obstruction
    a. Supraglottic: big tongue, foreign body
    b. Glottic: laryngeal spasm
    c. Subglottic: severe bronchospasm
2. Residual anesthesia
    a. Airway obstruction
    b. Volatile
    c. Narcotics
    d. Muscle relaxant
        - NDMR
            • Overdose
            • Inadequate reversal
            • Decreased metabolism or elimination
                a. Hypothermia
                b. Liver failure: pancuronium, rocuronium, vecuronium
                c. Kidney failure: pancuronium
            • Potentiation effect
                a. Neuromuscular diseases
                    i. Myasthenia gravis
                    ii. Muscular dystrophy (Duchenne)
                b. Drugs
                    i. Dantrolene
                    ii. Anesthetics: both volatile and local
                    iii. Ketamine
                    iv. Antibiotics (clindamycin, aminoglycosides)
                c. Electrolytes
                    i. Increased: Mg^{++}, Ca^{++}, lithium
                    ii. Decreased: K^{+}
        - Sux
            • Overdose – Type II block
            • Decreased pseudocholinesterase activity (also metabolizes ester local anesthetics and mivacurium)
                a. Atypical pseudocholinesterase (dibucaine 20% inhibition in homozygous)
                b. Hypothermia
                c. Drugs

           i.   Cholinesterase inhibitor
           ii. Pancuronium
           iii. Echothiophate
           iv. Reglan
           v.   Esmolol
   - Decreased pseudocholinesterase amount
           a. Liver disease
           b. Malnutrition
           c. Pregnancy
3. Vital: Hypocarbia, hypothermia
4. CNS complication

Hypoxia in Recovery Room

What do you think (differential)?
I think the most likely the cause in this case is ___, other differential includes:
1. Artifact
2. Airway obstruction
       a. Supra-glottic: big tongue, foreign body
       b. Glottis: laryngeal spasm
       c. Sub-glottic: severe bronchospasm
3. Respiratory drive depression
4. V/Q mismatch: atelectasis

PONV

IMPACT trial (NEJM 2004)

Risk factors (Each ↑ 20%):
1. Female
2. Non-smoker
3. h/o PONV
4. Post-op opioids
5. Hysterectomy /?cholecystectomy

Baseline risk:
   10% no risk factor
   20% 1 risk factor
   40% 2 risk factors
   60% 3 risk factors
   80% 4 risk factors

Intervention (Each ↓ 26%):
* Consider regional

1. Dexamethasone (4 mg, at the beginning of surgery, first line, effective for 24 h): ↓ 26%
2. TIVA (second line): ↓ 26%
    a. Propofol: ↓ 19%
    b. No nitrous oxide: ↓ 12%
3. Droperidol (1.25 mg) (no effect in male): ↓ 26%
4. Ondansetron (4 mg, reserved for rescue): ↓ 26%
5. Other anti-emetic medications
    a. Scopolamine patch
    b. Reglan: extrapyramidal SE
    c. Benadryl (25 mg)
    d. Phenergan (12.5 mg)

What do you think (differential)?
1. Risk factors for PONV
2. Vital
    a. Hypoxia
    b. Hypercarbia
    c. Hypotension
3. GI
    a. Obstruction
    b. Vagal stimulation

Delayed Emergence /Mental Status Change

What do you think (differential)?
I think the most likely the cause in this case is ___, other differential includes:
1. Anesthesia related
    a. Anesthetics
    b. Narcotics
    c. Neuromuscular blockers
    d. Other: sedative, benadryl, scopolamine…
    e. Hypothermia
2. Surgery related
    a. Surgical damage
    b. Stroke
3. Vital
    a. Hypotension
    b. Hypercarbia (CO_2 narcosis)
4. Neurological
    a. CVA (hemorrhagic, embolic, thrombotic)
    b. Cerebral edema
    c. Seizure
5. Metabolic
    a. DKA
    b. Hypoglycemia

What do you do? (Confirm, Vital, Rescue, Differential, Treatment)
1. Confirm: history (chart review), physical exam
2. Check
   a. ASA standard monitor
   b. Vt, airway pressure, breath sound bilateral
3. (Rescue)
4. Differential
   a. Medication
   b. Neurological: check pupil, ?CT, ?Neuro consult
   c. Lab: ABG, chem 7
5. Specific treatment

Agitation

What do you think (differential)?
I think the most likely the cause in this case is ___, other differential includes:
1. Anesthesia related
   a. Inadequate pain control
   b. Disorientation
   c. Bladder distension
   d. Medication: ketamine, steroid (steroid psychosis)
2. Vital
   a. Hypotension
   b. MI
   c. Hypoxia
   d. Hypercarbia
3. Neuro
   a. Parkinson's disease, reglan, droperidol
   b. Alcohol withdrawal
   c. Meningitis

What do you do?
1. Confirm: history (chart review), physical exam
2. Check
   a. ASA standard monitor
   b. Vt, breath sound bilateral
3. Rescue
4. Differential
   a. Labs: ABG, Chem7
   b. CXR
5. Specific treatment

Postop Fever

What do you think (differential)?

I think the most likely the cause in this case is ___, other differential includes:

1. Anesthesia related:
    a. MH
    b. Thyroid storm
    c. Atelectasis
2. Infection
    a. Wound infection
    b. UTI
    c. Sepsis

What do you do?

1. Confirm: history (chart review), physical exam
2. Vital
3. Rescue (Cooling measures)
    a. Remove blanket
    b. Cooled iv fluid
    c. Ice pack
    d. Tylenol
4. Differential
5. Specific treatment

Chapter 2 Preop Eval

General Preop Eval

1. Chart review
2. History
3. Physical exam
4. Lab
5. Specific tests

ASA Advisory for Preop Eval (2002)

Routine preoperative test in an asymptomatic patient is not recommended. Preoperative tests should be ordered on a selective basis for the purpose of guiding perioperative management.
1. ECG
    No specific minimum age for routine ECG
2. Cardiac eval
    2007 AHS advisory
3. CXR
    Extreme age, smoking, stable COPD, stable cardiac disease, resolved URI are not indication for CXR
4. H/H
    Routine H/H is not indicated
5. Chem 7
    Clinical characteristics should be considered before ordering

Preop Volume Access

1. History – I/O, weight loss, N/V, diarrhea
2. VS – Tachycardia, hypotension, weak pulse
3. Physical exam – Mucous membrane moisture, skin turgor, capillary refill, fontanelle, orthostatic hypotension (SBP drops 15 mmHg)
4. Lab – Hct, Na^+
5. Invasive monitor – CVP

HTN Preop Evaluation

1. Concerns about volume depletion, hemodynamic instability, and end organ dysfunction
2. Cancel elective surgery if DBP > 115 mmHg or SBP > 200 mmHg
3. Consider hold ACE inhibitor
4. A-line if pre-op BP is not controlled

5. Patient may have HTN during intubation and hypotension after induction
6. Keep intraop BP above 80% of preop level
7. Malignant HTN: 210/120 mmHg with encephalopathy and papilledema

Cardiovascular Eval for Noncardiac Surgery (2007 AHA Guidelines)

5 Steps
> Step 1 – Emergency surgery?
> Step 2 – Active cardiac condition?
> Step 3 – Low risk surgery?
> Step 4 – Cardiac function?
> Step 5 – Revised cardiac risk index

How would you do pre-op cardiovascular eval for noncardiac surgery?
1. Emergency surgery: go ahead
   a. Perioperative surveillance (e.g., serial ECGs, enzymes, monitoring)
   b. Risk reduction (e.g., beta-blockers with strict control of HR, statins, pain management).
2. Active cardiac condition: postpone elective surgery
   a. Acute MI (occurring within the past seven days)
   b. A *recent* MI (within the past eight to 30 days) with persistent symptoms or the results of stress testing
   c. Unstable or severe angina
   d. Decompensate heart failure
   e. Severe valvular disease (e.g., severe aortic stenosis)
   f. Significant arrhythmias (e.g., VT or Afib with a rapid rate)
   g. A recent MI without evidence of myocardium at risk – risk is equivalent to that of coronary artery disease (CAD).
3. Low-risk surgery: go ahead (for patients without active cardiac conditions)
4. Vascular, intermediate or high-risk procedures: assesses functional capacity.
   a. Asymptomatic patients with METs >4: go ahead
   b. Poor or indeterminate functional capacity: revised cardiac risk index
      - Ischemia heart disease
      - Heart failure
      - Cerebrovascular disease
      - DM
      - Renal Insufficiency
         • None - proceed to surgery
         • 3 or more - most likely to benefit from further testing only if it will change management.
         • 1 to 2 - proceeds to surgery with heart rate control or undergo noninvasive testing if it will change management.
         • *"There are insufficient data to determine the best strategy."*
         • Incidence of major cardiac events of 0.4%, 0.9%, 7% or 11% in patients with 0, 1, 2 or 3 risk predictors, respectively.

I.   Noninvasive stress testing and coronary revascularization before noncardiac surgery lack definitive benefits for risk reduction.
II.   Noncardiac surgery soon after revascularization (CABG or PCI with or without stents) is associated with high rates of perioperative morbidity and mortality.
III.   If revascularization is necessary, CABG or PCI without stenting or with a bare metal stent (BMS) should be considered.
IV.   Drug-eluting stents (DES) substantially impair arterial healing compared to BMS.
V.   Risk factors for CAD (e.g., smoking, family history, hypercholesterolemia, age and hypertension) have not been shown to predict perioperative cardiac morbidity.
VI.   In patients who need PCI and are likely to require invasive procedures within the next 12 months, consideration should be given to implantation of a BMS or balloon angioplasty alone instead of a DES.
VII.   There are potentially catastrophic risks of premature discontinuation of thienopyridine (e.g., clopidogrel or ticlopidine) therapy. The patient's cardiologist should be contacted to discuss optimal strategies of antiplatelet therapy.
VIII.   Neuraxial techniques (spinal and epidural) are not contraindicated in patients taking ASA, but are a concern in patients taking thienopyridine therapy. Clopidogrel therapy should be discontinued seven days before neuraxial blockade.

Coronary Artery Stent (ASA Practice Alert 2009, ACC/AHA Guidelines 2007)

What are your concerns about a recently placed coronary artery stent?
1. Dual antiplatelet therapy with ASA and thienopyridine (e.g., clopidogrel (plavix) or ticlopidine (ticlid)) is crucial to prevent stent thrombosis and MI
2. Minimum thienopyridine period for bare metal stent (BMS) is 4-6 weeks
3. Minimum thienopyridine period for drug-eluting stents (DES) is 12 months
4. Elective surgery should be postponed after the minimum thienopyridine treatment period
5. For emergent surgery, continue ASA, D/C thienopyridine, but resume thienopyridine ASAP
6. Bridging thienopyridine with coumadin, antithrombotics, or glycoprotein IIb/IIIa agents has no benefit.

Endocarditis Prophylaxis (2007 AHA Guidelines)

Conditions that need prophylaxis
1. Prosthetic cardiac valve
2. h/o endocarditis
3. Unrepaired cyanotic congenital heart disease
4. Repaired congenital heart disease with prosthetic material or device
5. Cardiac transplantation recipients with cardiac valvular disease

Antibiotic
1. Ampicillin 2G (50 mg/kg pedi) or cefazolin / ceftriaxone 1G (50 mg/kg pedi) IV

2. Clindamycin 600 mg (20 mg/kg pedi) or cefazolin / ceftriaxone 1G (50 mg/kg pedi) IV if allergic to PCN

- No longer recommended for patients who undergo a GI or GU tract procedure, including patients with the highest risk

Periop Management of Pacemakers & ICDs (ASA 2005 Advisory)

1. Preoperative Evaluation
   a. Establish if pt has a pacer/ICD
   b. Define the type of pacer/ICD
   c. Whether pt is pacer dependent
   d. Determine pacer/ICD's response to magnet
2. Preoperative Preparation
   a. Determine if there is anything intra-op that might interfere with pacer/ICD (electrocautery, radiofrequency, lithotripsy, MRI, ECT or radiation)
   b. Temporary pacing and defibrillation equipment should be immediately available
   c. Suspend defibrillation function with magnet or programming
   d. Suggest surgeon to use bipolar electrocautery
   e. Electrocautery grounding plate at a position where the current pathway does not pass through pacer/ICD
3. Intraoperative Management
   a. Use bipolar is possible
   b. Use electrocautery at short intermittent bursts at lowest feasible energy level
   c. Intraop VT or Vfib that needs defibrillation of cardioversion
      - Stop surgery
      - Remove magnet to enable antitachycardia therapy
      - Emergency external defibrillation or cardioversion if ICD doesn't work
         - Place paddles as far as possible from pulse generator
         - Use a clinically appropriate energy output
4. Postoperative Management
   a. Temporary pacing and defibrillation equipment should be immediately available
   b. Continue monitor
   c. Interrogate and restore pacer/ICD function

Pacemaker/ICD Code

Pacemaker Code
1. Pacing chamber (O, A, V, D)
2. Sensing chamber (O, A, V, D)
3. Response to sensing (O, I, T, D)

4. Programmability (O, R)
5. Multisite pacing (O, A, V, D)

Defibrillator Code
1. Shock chamber (O, A, V, D)
2. Antitachycardia pacing chamber (O, A, V, D)
3. Tachycardia detection (Electrogram, Hemodynamic)
4. Antibradycardia pacing chamber (O, A, V, D)

Preop Cardiac Tests

1. Treadmill stress test
2. Dobutamine stress echocardiography
    a. Regional wall abnormality
    b. Avoid dobutamine in tachy patients
3. Persantine thallium imaging
    a. Perfusion deficits
    b. Avoid persantine in asthma /severe COPD patients
4. Coronary angiography

ASA Classification

- Class I: Normal healthy patient
- Class II: Patient with mild systemic disease (no functional limitation)
- Class III: Patient with severe systemic disease (some functional limitation)
- Class IV: Patient with severe systemic disease as constant threat to life
- Class V: Pt is not expected to survive without surgery
- Class VI: Brain-dead patient for organ removal
- E: Emergency surgery

Chapter 3 Regional Anesthesia

Advantage of Regional Anesthesia

1. Avoid airway problems
2. Reduce incidence of PONV
3. Better postop pain control
4. Might avoid periop narcotics
5. Might reduce incidence of DVT and PE

in trauma
— Assuming there is no
evidence of coagulopathy
by H&P and

Absolute Contraindications to Neuraxial Blockade

1. Coagulopathy or thrombocytopenia
2. Severe hypotension or hypovolemia
3. Severe aortic stenosis
4. Severe mitral stenosis
5. Intracranial hypertension
6. Patient refuses
7. Infection at insertion site

Factors Influence the Spread of Spinal Anesthesia

1. Baricity of anesthetic solution
   a. Add glucose to make hyperbaric
   b. Add water to make hypobaric
2. Position of the patient
   a. In supine position, T6 is the lowest, and L3 is the highest
3. Drug dosage
   a. The higher the dosage, the higher the level

- Needle insertion site: ~ L4-5 to avoid spinal cord, which ends ~ L1 in adult

Complications of Neuraxial Anesthesia

Complications associated with medication injection
1. Inadequate anesthesia or analgesia
2. Total spinal anesthesia
   a. Unconsciousness, apnea, and hypotension from high level of spinal anesthesia
   b. Rapid onset
   c. ABC to rescue
   d. Apnea is often transient

     e. Prevented with aspiration before injection, testing dose, and injection with incremental doses

3. Subdural injection
     a. Symptoms similar to high spinal anesthesia
     b. Slow onset
     c. Supportive treatment

4. Intravascular injection
     a. Prevented with aspiration before injection, testing dose, and injection with incremental doses
     b. 1:200,000 (5 μg/ml) epinephrine
     c. HR increase 20% or T wave amplitude increase 25% indicates intravascular injection (when epi is added)
     d. Bupivacaine is the most toxic and chloroprocaine is the least toxic
     e. Amiodarone and lipid infusion for bupivacaine induced arrhythmia

5. Sympathetic block
     a. Hypotension
     b. Bradycardia and cardiac arrest (T1-T4 level blockade)

6. Urinary retention
     a. Foley should be used in all neuraxial anesthesia pt

Complications associated with needle insertion
1. Postdural puncture headache
2. Epidural or spinal hematoma
3. Epidural abscess
     a. Around 5 days from epidural cath insertion
     b. Normally remove epidural cath in 4 days
     c. MRI/CT to confirm
     d. Treatment: surgical decompression, antibiotics, perQ drainage
4. Sheering of epidural catheter
     a. Observe if cath is deep in tissue
     b. Remove cath if it is superficial to prevent infection
5. Neurological injury: intra spinal cord injection causes paraplegia

Postdural Puncture Headache (PDPH)

Symptoms
1. Characteristic positional headache
2. Can have diplopia and tinnitus
3. Onset is normally hours after procedure, but can happen immediately
4. Can follow seemingly uncomplicated epidural

Pathophysiology
    CSF loss causing traction of the structures that supports the brain

Risk factors
1. Young age

2. Female
3. Pregnancy
4. Large needle
5. Cutting point needle

Treatment
1. Bed rest
2. Hydration (stimulates CSF production)
3. Analgesia (tylenol, NSAIDs)
4. Caffeine (stimulates CSF production)
5. Fioricet (tylenol, caffeine, a barbiturate (butalbital))
6. Blood patch
   a. Can be effective immediately or in a few hours
   b. Most patient response to single blood patch
   c. Can try 2nd blood patch if 1st one is not effective
   d. Prophylactic blood patch is controversial

Epidural Hematoma

Risk factors
1. Insertion and removal of epidural cath
2. Abnormal coagulation or bleeding disorders

Symptoms
1. Sharp back pain and leg pain
2. Neurological deficits
   a. Numbness or weakness of legs
   b. Urinary or bowel incontinence
3. More sudden onset compared with epidural abscess

Management
1. Immediate MRI if suspected
2. Need surgical decompression within 8 hours

Regional Anesthesia in Anticoagulated Patients
(2002 ASRA Consensus Statements)

1. Unfractionated Heparin
   a. Pre-op SQ (mini dose for prophylaxis)
      - No risk
      - Check plt if on heparin > 4d to rule out HIT
   b. Intra-op IV (vascular case)
      - Administer at least 1 h after needle placement
      - Remove cath 2 h after last dose if PTT <35
      - Resume 1 h after cath removal

- Bloody/difficult placement is not an indication to cancel case
  c. Intra-op IV (cardiac case)
    - Insufficient data to determine if it is risky
2. LMWH (lovenox – enoxaparin)
   a. Pre-op
     - Thromboprophylaxis dose (< 60 mg QD)
       • Wait 10-12 h before needle placement
     - Therapeutic dose (1 mg/kg Q12h or 1.5 mg/kg QD)
       • Wait 24 h before needle placement
   b. Post-op
     - QD dose (< 60 mg QD)
       • 1st dose 6-8 h post-op
       • 2nd dose 24 h after 1st dose
       • Remove cath 10-12 h after last dose
       • Resume 2 h after removal
     - BID dose
       • 1st dose 24 h post-op
       • Remove cath before 1st dose
       • Start 2 h after removal
3. Coumadin
   a. Pre-op
     - Check INR if treatment > 24h or more than 1 dose (INR < 1.4)
     - Stop 4-5 days & INR < 1.4
   b. Post-op
     - Remove cath if INR < 1.5
     - Resume on the same day of cath removal
4. Antiplatelet Medications
   a. NSAIDs/ASA: no risk
   b. Plavix (clopidogrel)
     - Pre-op
       • Stop 7 days
     - Post-op
       • Wait 7 days to remove cath
       • Resume 24 h after removal
5. Thrombolytic therapy: no definite recommendation
6. Herbs: no risk

Complications of Interscalene Block

Needle tip location
1. Intravascular, particularly vertebral artery injection
2. Epidural, subdural, spinal
3. PTX

Medication spread

1. Stellate ganglion block
   a. Horner's syndrome: myosis, ptosis, enophthalmos, anhidrosis
2. Phrenic nerve block
3. Recurrent laryngeal nerve block

Bier Block

1. 2 tourniquets. Inflate the proximal one first. 30 min later deflate the proximal one and inflate the distal one for another 20 min
2. Keep tourniquet up for at least 15 min after lidocaine injection

Ankle Block

Superficial peroneal, deep peroneal, saphenous, posterior tibial, and sural nerves

Chapter 4 Respiratory

Possible Nerve Blocks for Awake FOI

1. Glossopharyngeal nerve – palatoglossal arch
2. Superior laryngeal nerve – 1 cm below greater cornu of hyoid bone
3. Recurrent laryngeal nerve (intratracheal block) – 4% lidocaine at end expiration
4. CN V (nasal) – 4% lidocaine with 0.25% phenylephrine

Obstructive Sleep Apnea (ASA Guidelines 2006)

Pre-op eval
1. Chart review, H&P, CPAP/BiPAP?
2. Sleep study?

Intra-op
1. Regional is preferred
2. Anticipate difficult airway
3. Extubate when fully awake

Asthma

Preop considerations
1. History –hospitalized for asthma? Taking steroids?
2. Physical exam – wheezing, pulsus paradoxus
3. ABG – normal or hypercarbia indicates severe disease in acute attack
4. PFTs – FEV_1/FVC (normal > 80%), $FEF_{25-75\%}$ (forced mid expiratory flow)
5. Consider hydrocortisone 100 mg q8h if pt is on chronic steroids
6. Consider avoiding ranitidine because unopposed H1 activity may make asthma worse

Treatment
1. β2 agonist – albuterol
2. Glucocorticoids
3. Anticholinergic – ipratropium
4. Mast cell stabilizer – cromolyn
5. Phosphodiesterase inhibitor – Theophylline (narrow therapeutic window)
   a. Theophylline toxicity: tachycardia, arrhythmia, CNS excitation, nausea, diarrhea

Anesthesia considerations
1. Ketamine produces bronchial dilation and is the induction agent of choice in actively wheezing patient
   a. Ketamine with theophylline causes seizure

2. Propofol is also a good induction agent for asthma pt
3. Volatiles are potent bronchodilator
4. Avoid histamine release medications (morphine, meperidine)
5. Monitor capnography wave form
6. Consider deep extubation

COPD

Anesthesia considerations
1. PFTs: FEV_1, FEV_1/FVC, FEF_{25-75}
2. Cardiac: chronic hypoxia causes pulm HTN and RV failure
3. Risk of PTX because of bullae
4. Avoid N_2O if pulm HTN or bullae

Airway Obstruction

Acute epiglottitis
1. Clinical features
   a. Sudden onset of fever, stridor, drooling, hoarseness, chest retraction, sitting position
   b. Total airway obstruction can happen anytime
   c. ET tube and antibiotics are life saving
   d. Thumb-like epiglottic shadow on lateral view
   e. Bacterial infection, esp. H influenzae
   f. Becoming more common in adult
2. Anesthesia concerns
   a. Inhalational induction in sitting position with small ET tube
   b. No DL before induction because of possible laryngospasm
   c. Ready for tracheostomy before induction
   d. Inhalational induction in sitting position in OR
   e. Small ET tube
   f. IV line or radiology studies are not necessary before induction

Infectious Croup
1. Clinical features
   a. Barking cough
   b. Usually follows URTI
   c. Subglottic obstruction – Staple sign
   d. Usually do not need intubation
2. Anesthesia concerns
   a. Treat with racemic epinephrine nebulizer and decadron iv
   b. Intubate in severe case

Foreign Body

1. Clinical features
    a. Stridor – supraglottic and glottic obstruction
    b. Wheezing – subglottic obstruction
    c. May not have clear aspiration history
2. Anesthesia concerns
    a. Airway manipulation may change partial obstruction into complete obstruction
        -   Ready for tracheostomy before induction
        -   Inhalational induction
        -   DL or bronchoscopy to remove foreign body

Laryngeal Polyps

Anesthesia concerns
1. No preop sedation if severe airway obstruction
2. Inhalation induction if severe airway obstruction
3. CO_2 laser can cause corneal injury (special glasses)
4. Vaporized debris are hazardous to OR personnel (special mask)

Ventilation
1. Through small ET tube
    a. Helium has less density and easier to pass small ET tube (turbulent flow)
    b. Most common helium-oxygen mixtures are 80%/20% and 70%/30%
2. Intermittent apnea technique
3. Venturi jet ventilation
    a. Inspiration
        -   1-2 seconds
        -   High flow O_2 sucks room air into lung
    b. Expiration
        -   Need longer time (4-6 seconds) for exhalation to avoid barotrauma
        -   Crucial to monitor chest wall movement
    c. Complications: barotrauma, gastric dilation
4. High-frequency jet ventilation
    a. Initial setting
        -   Rate of 120-240 breaths/min
        -   Inspiratory time of 33%
        -   Drive pressure of 15-30 psi
        -   Mean airway pressure measured at least 5 cm distal to injector
    b. Oxygenation is proportional to mean airway pressure
    c. CO_2 elimination is proportional to drive pressure

Prevention of laser related airway fire
1. Specific ET tube
    a. Polyvinylchloride tubes – release HCl when ignited
    b. Red rubber tubes – release black smoke when ignited
    c. Metal tubes
    d. Metallic tape

2. ET tube cuff filled with NS and methylene blue
3. FiO$_2$ as low as possible ($\leq$ 30%), no N$_2$O
4. Saline soaked pledgets in airway to reduce risk
5. Water (60 ml syringe) immediately available

Management of airway fire (ASA Advisory 2008)
1. Extinguish fire
    a. Immediately remove ET tube
    b. Stop all airway gases
    c. Remove sponges and any other flammable materials from airway
    d. Pour saline into airway
2. Ventilation
    a. Once fire is out, re-establish ventilation
    b. No N$_2$O, low FiO$_2$
3. Exam damage
    a. Exam ET tube to see if fragments may be left in airway
    b. Consider bronchoscopy
    c. Consider bronchial lavage and steroids

Management of non-airway OR fire (ASA Advisory 2008)
1. Extinguish fire
    a. Immediately stop all airway gases
    b. Remove drapes and all burning and flammable materials
    c. Extinguish burning materials by pouring saline
2. Re-establish ventilation
    a. Once fire is out, maintain ventilation
3. Exam damage
    a. Assess for inhalation injury if pt is not intubated

Mediastinal Mass

Preop eval
1. Airway obstruction
    a. History
        - Dyspnea, nonproductive cough
        - Airway obstruction worse when lying down (pt prefers upright position)
        - Asymptomatic pt can develop severe airway obstruction after induction
    b. Physical exam: Tracheal deviation, wheezing
    c. CT scan
    d. Flow-volume loops
        - Extrathoracic variable obstruction – flat Inspiration curve
        - Intrathoracic variable obstruction – flat Expiration curve
        - Fixed large obstruction – flat both inspiration and expiration curve
2. Superior vena cava syndrome

    a.   Reduced preload with severely decreased CO

    b.   Edema of head, neck, and arm

    c.   Can have heart compression and/or pericardial infusion from invasion

    d.   Asymptomatic pt can develop cardiac collapse after induction

Anesthesia concerns
1. Local anesthesia if possible and indicated
2. Preop radiation or chemo if possible to shrink mass
3. No premed
4. Transfer pt in sitting position
5. Large-bore iv in lower extremity
6. A-line
7. Awake FOI first choice
8. Inhalation induction in uncooperative pt
9. No muscle relaxant before a reliable airway is established
10. Can have severe induction related complications in pt without preop airway compression or superior vena cava syndrome
11. Positive-pressure ventilation can cause severe hypotension
12. Extubate only when pt is fully awake with an air leak around ET tube

Complication of mediastinoscopy
1. PTX
2. Vessel Damage
   a. Excessive hemorrhage
   b. Air embolism
3. Vessel Compression
   a. Loss pulse of right arm (right subclavian A. compression)
   b. Bradycardia (trachea or vagus N. compression)
   c. Stroke (innominate A. compression)
4. Nerve Damage
   a. Recurrent laryngeal nerve
   b. Phrenic nerve

Tracheal Resection

Anesthesia considerations
1. No premed
2. A-line for possible big vessel injury
3. Inhalation induction with 100% O_2 and sevoflurane
4. No muscle relaxant
5. Rigid bronchoscopy by surgeon
   a. Ventilation through side arm of rigid bronchoscopy
   b. Apneic oxygenation
   c. Jet vent
6. Postop neck flexion to reduce suture tension

Tonsillectomy and Adenoidectomy

Pre-op
1. Assess airway and apnea
2. No sedation for pt with severe obstruction or apnea

Intraop
1. Inhalation induction without muscle relaxant in severe obstructive pt
2. Cuffed ET tube
3. Stomach suction before extubation
4. Extubate after fully awake with head turn to the side

Postop
1. Nausea is common
2. Child < 3 yr old is admitted overnight for possible bleeding and airway obstruction
3. For post-op bleeding tonsil, volume resuscitation is essential
4. RSI after NG tube suction for reoperation to control bleeding

One Lung Ventilation

Indication for one-lung ventilation
1. Restrict disease to one lung
    a. Infection
    b. Bleeding
2. Restrict ventilation to one lung
    a. Large lung bulla
    b. Bronchopleural fistula
3. Surgery exposure:
    a. Lung surgeries
    b. Esophageal surgeries
    c. Aortic aneurysm repair

Physiology
1. Right-to-left intrapulmonary shunt results in hypoxia
2. Blood flow to nonventilated lung is decreased by hypoxic pulmonary vasoconstriction
3. Inhibition of hypoxic pulmonary vasoconstriction increases shunting
    a. Vasodilators (nitroglycerin, nitroprusside)
    b. Volatile anesthetics
    c. Pneumonia
    d. Hypocarbia
4. Reducing blood flow to ventilated lung also ↑ shunting
    a. Low FiO_2
    b. High mean airway pressure
    c. Vasoconstriction
5. Little effect on CO_2 elimination

Major difference between right and left main bronchi
1. Diverge angle: 25 degree for right bronchus, 45 degree for left bronchus
2. Lob branches: 3 (upper, middle, and lower) for right bronchus, 2 (upper and lower) for left bronchus
3. Distance between upper lobe orifice and carina: 2 cm for right bronchus, 5 cm for left bronchus

Techniques
1. Double-lumen tube
   a. Left sided double-lumen tube
      - The most commonly used double-lumen tube
   b. Right sided double-lumen tube
      - Opening in bronchial cuff for right upper lobe ventilation
      - More difficult to place
   c. Blue balloon is for Blue cuff at Bronchial lumen
      - Careful in inflation to avoid bronchial rupture
   d. Position confirmation with fiberoptic bronchoscope
      - Through tracheal lumen
        • Carina must be visible
        • Bronchial lumen should be in the correct bronchus
        • Bronchial cuff should be just visible in the correct bronchus
      - Through bronchial lumen
        • Critical for right-side double-lumen tube
          a. Make sure the opening in bronchial cuff is at the orifice of right upper lobe
      - Reposition under fiberoptic bronchoscope guidance if the bronchial lumen is in the wrong bronchus
      - Reconfirm the tube position whenever pt's position is changed
   e. Might need to change to single-lumen tube if pt needs post-op ventilation
2. Single-lumen tube with bronchial block
3. Single-lumen bronchial tube

Complications of double-lumen tubes
1. Tube misplacement leading to hypoxia
2. Laryngitis
3. Bronchial rupture from bronchial cuff overinflation

Management of hypoxia during OLV (as the following order)
1. Increase FiO_2
2. Change vent setting such Vt and RR (limited effect)
3. Low PEEP to ventilated lung (might worsen hypoxia by reducing blood flow to ventilated lung)
4. Reinflate the collapsed lung (might intervene surgery)
5. CPAP to the collapsed lung (very effective but intervene surgery)
6. Clamp or ligate PA of the collapsed lung
7. Convert to two lung ventilation

ARDS

Definition
1. Acute onset
2. Bilateral infiltrate
3. Wedge pressure < 18 mmHg or clinically lack evidence of LV dysfunction
4. ARDS if $PaO_2/FiO_2 < 200$
5. ALI if $PaO_2/FiO_2 < 300$

Treatment
1. Low Vt of 6 ml/kg (NEJM 2000, ARDS Network)
2. Low PEEP (8 cmH_2O) has the same clinical outcome as high PEEP (13 cmH_2O)
3. Conservative fluid management (NEJM 2006)
4. Steroid has no benefit (NEJM 2006)

Risk Factors for Postop Pulmonary Complications

1. Preop lung disease
2. Thoracic and upper abdominal surgery
3. Smoking
4. Obesity
5. > 60 yo
   - Stop smoking for > 6 wks to resume pulmonary function
   - Stop smoking for 1 day is also beneficial to reduce CO level

Ventilation Mode in ICU

1. CMV – continuous mandatory ventilation
   a. The most commonly used mode in ICU
   b. Fixed Vt and rate regardless of pt's effort
2. IMV – intermittent mandatory ventilation
   a. Fixed Vt
   b. Allows spontaneous ventilation
   c. SIMV – synchronized intermittent mandatory ventilation
      - Mechanical ventilation is synchronized with spontaneous ventilation
3. PSV – positive pressure ventilation
   a. Pt's spontaneous breathing triggers ventilator to deliver a positive pressure to assist Vt
   b. Usually needs low frequency IMV to back up for safety
4. PEEP – positive end-expiratory pressure
   a. Prevents atelectasis and improves oxygenation
   b. Usually 5-20 cmH_2O

Hb-O₂ Dissociation Curve

Factors move curve to right (everything ↑)
1. ↑ P_{50}
2. Acidosis (↑ H^+)
3. ↑ Temperature
4. ↑ 2,3 DPG
5. ↑ CO_2 level
6. Pregnancy
7. HbS

Factors move curve to left (everything ↓)
1. ↓ P_{50}
2. Alkalosis (↓ H^+)
3. ↓ Temperature
4. ↓ 2,3 DPG
5. ↓ CO_2 level
6. HbF
7. COHb
8. Methemoglobinemia

Equations

1. O_2 content $= (1.31 \times SO_2 \times Hb) + (0.003 \times PO_2)$
2. $P_IO_2 = (760 - PH_2O) \times FiO_2$
3. $P_AO_2 = P_IO_2 - PaCO_2/0.8$

Side Effect of O₂ Therapy

1. Lung toxicity (100% for up to 10 h is OK)
2. Absorption atelectasis
3. Retinopathy of prematurity
4. Fire hazard
5. Respiratory depression in COPD (spont. breathing)

Chapter 5 Cardiac

ECG

- Lead II for P wave and inferior wall ischemia
- Lead V5 for anterior wall ischemia
- V5 if only one channel can be monitored
- ST depression (especially down-sloping and horizontal) – endocardial injury
- ST elevation – epicardial injury
- Peak T wave – endocardial ischemia
- Reverse T wave – epicardial ischemia
- II, III, aVF: inferior wall – RCA
- V5: anterior wall – LAD
- I, aVL: lateral wall – CX
- SA node – RCA or LAD
- AV node – RCA
- Small ST elevation in V3 and V4 is normal in young patients

PA Catheter

Complications
1. Needle insertion related
   a. Hematoma
   b. Air embolism
   c. PTX
2. Cath insertion related
   a. RBBB
   b. Arrhythmia
3. Cath related
   a. PA perforation
   b. Balloon rupture
   c. Thrombosis
   d. Infection

Wedge pressure vs. LVEDP
1. Wedge pressure > LVEDP
   a. MS
   b. High airway pressure
2. Wedge pressure < LVEDP
   a. AR
   b. Stiff LV

Relative Contraindication

1. LBBB
2. WPW
   a. Need PAC with pacing capability

Cardiac Stroke Volume Determinants

1. Preload
   a. LV End-diastolic volume
   b. Starling law
   c. Atrial contraction contributes 20% ventricular filling
   d. LVEDP to estimate preload only with normal ventricular compliance
      - LV compliance is reduced in LVH, ischemia, and pericarditis
2. Pump
   a. Contractility
   b. Wall motion abnormality
   c. Valvular function
   d. Normal EF 50-65%
3. Afterload
   a. LV systolic wall tension or arterial impedance to injection
   b. $SVR = 80 \times (MAP - CVP)/CO$ (normal 900-1500 $dyn.s.cm^{-5}$)

Determinants of Myocardial O₂ Supply and Consumption

O_2 Supply
   1. HR
      a. Diastolic time
   2. Coronary perfusion pressure
      a. Difference between aortic pressure and ventricular pressure
      b. LV is perfused during diastole
      c. RV is perfused both systole and diastole
   3. Patency of coronary arteries
   4. Arterial oxygen content

O_2 Consumption
   1. HR
   2. Wall tension
      a. Preload
      b. Afterload
   3. Contractility

Cardiovascular Agents

Adrenergic Agonist

1. Phenylephrine
    a. Mainly α1 agonist
    b. ↑ BP, ↓ CO and HR
2. Norepinephrine
    a. All except β2
    b. ↑ BP, minor change in HR and CO
3. Ephedrine
    a. Indirect and direct, all receptors
    b. ↑ BP, HR, and CO
4. Epinephrine
    a. All receptors
    b. One of the most potent inotropes
    c. ↑ BP, HR, CO
5. Dobutamine
    a. β1 agonist
    b. ↑ CO, minor change in BP and HR
6. Dopamine
    a. DA1/DA2 (< 2 mcg/kg/min)
    b. β1 (2-10 mcg/kg/min)
    c. α1 (> 10 mcg/kg/min)
    d. ↑ CO, BP, HR
7. Isoproterenol
    a. β1 and β2 agonist
    b. ↑ CO and HR, ↓ BP
8. Fenoldopam
    a. DA1 agonist
    b. ↓ BP, ↑ HR, no change in CO
9. Dexmedetomidine
    a. α2 agonist (α1 also on high dose)
    b. Sedative and sympatholytic effects that blunt many of the cardiovascular response during periop period, with minimal respiratory depression
    c. HTN if rapid administration, hypotension and bradycardia during ongoing therapy
10. Clonidine
    a. α2 agonist
    b. Antihypertensive
    c. Side effects: respiratory depression, bradycardia, sedation, dry mouth
11. Methyldopa
    a. α2 > α1
    b. Treat HTN in pregnancy

Phosphodiesterase III inhibitors
1. Milrinone
    a. Inotrope without increase myocardial oxygen consumption
    b. ↑ CO, minor change in HR, ↓ BP
    c. ↓ PVR
2. Amrinone

    a.   Associated with thrombocytopenia

Vasopressin
    a.   V1 agonist
    b.   Equivalent to epinephrine in Vfib and PEA
    c.   Also used in septic shock

Hypotensive Agents
1. Adrenergic Antagonist
    a.   Labetalol – blocks $\alpha1$, $\beta1$, $\beta2$
    b.   Phenoxybenzamine PO – blocks $\alpha1$
    c.   Phentolamine iv – blocks $\alpha1$
    d.   Esmolol /metoprolol – block $\beta1$
    e.   Propranolol – block $\beta1$ & $\beta2$
2. Nitroprusside
    a.   Effect on Organ Systems
     - Cardiac
       • ↓ Preload > ↓ afterload
       • Coronary artery dilation may result in coronary steal phenomenon
     - Respiratory
       • ↓ Pulmonary artery pressure
       • ↑ V/Q mismatch and shunt
     - Cerebral
       • Dilate cerebral vessel and ↑ CBF
     - Renal
       • Renal function maintained despite ↓ BP and renal perfusion
    b.   Cyanide toxicity
     - Physiology
       • Interfere with tissue O_2 utilization
       • Rare with cumulative dose < 0.5 mg/kg/h
     - Signs
       • Tachyphylaxis
       • Metabolic acidosis
       • ↑ Venous oxygen content
       • Arrhythmia
     - Treatment
       • 100% O_2
       • Sodium thiosulfate
       • Sodium nitrate
    c.   Methemoglobinemia
     - Signs
       • Pulse oximeter reading remains at 85% regardless of SaO_2
     - Treatment:
       • Methylene blue
     - Other causes

- Prilocaine and benzocaine
    d. General Information
        - Metabolized to nitric oxide to activate cGMP
        - 100 mcg/ml solution protected from light, 0.5-10 mcg/kg/min
3. Nitroglycerin
    a. Effect on Organ Systems
        - Cardiac
            • ↓ Preload > ↓ afterload
            • Redistribute coronary blood to ischemia area, no coronary steal
        - Respiratory
            • Relax bronchial smooth muscle
            • ↓ Pulmonary artery pressure
            • ↑ V/Q mismatch and shunt
        - Cerebral
            • Dilate cerebral vessel and ↑ CBF
            • HA
        - Other
            • Uterine relaxation
    b. Methemoglobinemia – rare
    c. General Information
        - Metabolized to nitric oxide to activate cGMP
        - 100 mcg/ml solution in glass container & specific tubing, 0.5-10 mcg/kg/min
4. Hydralazine
    a. ↓ Afterload, potent cerebral vasodilator
    b. Often used in preeclampsia
5. Fenoldopam
    a. Avoid in asthma and sulfa allergy patients

Arrhythmia

AV block
- 1st degree: PR interval > 0.2 s
- 2nd degree type I: progressive prolongation of PR interval till a P wave is not conducted
- 2nd degree type II: P wave is not conducted without progressive PR interval prolongation
- 3rd degree: complete AV dissociation

Indication for temporary pacer:
1. Symptomatic bradycardia
2. MI with new BBB, type II 2nd degree block, or 3rd block
3. Bifascicular block in coma patient

Temporary pacing methods

1. Transcutaneous
2. Transvenous
3. Transesophageal
4. Epicardial

Antiarrhythmic agents
- Class I: sodium channel blockers – lidocaine, procainamide
- Class II: β blockers
- Class III: amiodarone (amiodarone has character of multiple classes)
- Class IV: Ca channel blockers
- Class V: digoxin

WPW Syndrome
1. PR interval < 0.12 s, δ wave in QRS complex
2. Avoid factors that cause sympathetic stimulation
   a. Pretreatment with β blockers
   b. Avoid ketamine and pancuronium, cautious for anticholinergics
   c. Intubation only after pt is deeply anesthetized
3. Adenosine is the drug of choice for PSVT
4. Procainamide, amiodarone and β blockers for treatment
5. Avoid digoxin and verapamil because they decrease AV node conduction

Valvular Diseases

Aortic Stenosis
1. Normal area 2.5-3.5 cm^2
2. Severe AS: area < 0.7 cm^2, gradient > 50 mmHg
3. Clinical symptoms: trial of dyspnea on exertion, angina, syncope
4. Fixed stroke volume, CO is HR dependent
5. Hemodynamic goal: relatively high BP, relatively high HR (60-90), keep sinus rhythm

Mitral Stenosis
1. Normal 4-6 cm^2
2. Critical MS: area < 1.0 cm^2, gradient > 20 mmHg
3. Hemodynamic goal: relatively high BP; relatively low HR, keep sinus rhythm

Mitral Valve Prolapse
1. High incidence in scoliosis and Marfan syndrome
2. Associated with sudden death
3. Hemodynamic goal: relatively high BP; relatively low HR

Hypertrophic Cardiomyopathy (HOCM)
1. Associated with sudden death
2. Treat with β blocker to reduce contractility
3. Hemodynamic goal: relatively high BP; relatively low HR

Aortic Regurgitation
1. Severe AR: regurgitation fraction > 60% of stroke volume
2. EF does not represent effective stroke volume
3. Hemodynamic goal: relatively low BP, relative high HR (80-100)

Mitral Regurgitation
1. Severe MR: regurgitation fraction > 60% of stroke volume
2. EF does not represent effective stroke volume
3. Hemodynamic goal: relatively low BP, relative high HR (80-100)

Tricuspid Regurgitation
1. Hemodynamic goal: avoid pulm HTN
2. Issues with PAC
   a. Difficult to flow
   b. CO falsely elevated with thermodilution method

Tetralogy of Fallot
1. Maintain systemic BP and reduce pulm BP to avoid right-to-left shunt
2. Induce with ketamine
3. Right-to-left shunt causes slow inhalation induction but fast iv induction
4. Surgical treatment: Blalock-Taussig (left subclavian to pulm artery) shunt

General Rules of Hemodynamic Goal for Valvular Disease (AS, MS, HOCM, MVP, AR, MR)
1. Keep BP relatively high in all valvular diseases, including tamponade, except in regurgitation diseases.
2. In general the goal for HR is in opposite to the goal for BP, except in AS, which both BP and HR should be high

Cardiac Tamponade

Pathophysiology
1. Reduced and fixed preload
2. CO is rate dependent
3. Equalization of diastolic pressure: RAP = RVEDP = LAP = LVEDP

Signs and symptoms
1. Hypotension, tachycardia, tachypnea
2. Muffled heart sound, jugular distension
3. Pulsus paradoxus (SBP drops 10 mmHg in inspiration)
4. EKG: diffuse low voltage, electrical alternans, generalized ST elevation
5. Diagnosed with 2D echo
6. Pericardiocentesis can be life saving

Anesthesia concerns
1. Goal is to keep BP and HR relative high (as AS)

2. Pt is prepped and draped, and surgeons are ready before induction
3. Ketamine and pancuronium are induction agents
4. Maintain with ketamine till tamponade is relieved
5. Avoid vigorous positive-pressure ventilation before chest is opened
6. Epinephrine as inotrope and chronotrope
7. Watch for bradycardia during pericardial manipulation

Cardiac Anesthesia

Components of Cardiopulmonary Bypass (CPB) Circuit
1. Venous reservoir
    a. Fluid level is critical to prevent air embolism
2. Oxygenator
3. Heat exchanger
4. Pump
    a. Roller pump
        - Constant flow regardless resistance
        - Can provide pulsatile flow
    b. Centrifugal pump
        - Less RBC damage
        - Does not pump air bubbles
        - Flow is afterload dependent
5. Filters

Hypothermia
1. ~ 32 °C for regular CPB
2. ~ 17 °C for total circulatory arrest
3. For each ↓ 10 °C, ↓ O_2 consumption 50%

Cardioplegia
1. High K^+
2. ~ 15 °C
3. Arrest in diastole
4. Repeat q30 min because of rewarming and washout

Anesthesia Technique
1. IV induction with volatile maintenance
    a. Etomidate or propofol (1 mg/kg) for induction
    b. Rocuronium and vecuronium for relaxant. Sux for RSI.
        - Vecuronium may enhance opioid-induced bradycardia
        - Pancuronium if bradycardia
    c. Total dose of fentanyl <15 mcg/kg for fast track
    d. Iso, sevo, des are all OK for maintenance
2. TIVA
3. High-dose opioid anesthesia
    a. Prolonged postop respiratory depression

      b.   High incidence of intraop awareness
4.   Neuraxial anesthesia is not popular in US in concern of epidural hematoma

Cannulation
1.   Aortic cannulation
      a.   Keep SBP ~ 100 mmHg
2.   Venous cannulation
      a.   Single cannula with 2 ports (one in RA and one in IVC) for CABG and AVR
      b.   Two cannulas (one in SVC and one in IVC) for open heart surgery
      c.   Hold breath during RA incision to prevent air embolism
      d.   Watch for A-fib and hypotension
3.   Retrograde cardioplegia cath placement
      a.   In coronary sinus
4.   LV vent
      a.   Through pulm vein
      b.   Reduce LV tension and O_2 consumption
      c.   Blood from bronchial, pleural and thebesian veins
5.   Antegrade cardioplegia cath placement
      a.   Through aortic root, coronary ostia, or graft

Anticoagulation and Bleeding Prophylaxis
1.   Heparin
      a.   Activates antithrombin III 1000 fold
      b.   ~ 3.5 mg/kg through central line before CPB, 5 mg/kg if pt on preop heparin gtt
      c.   Check ACT (activated coagulation time) 3-5 min after (lineal relationship between ACT and heparin dosage)
      d.   If ACT < 450 (480 at some centers), add another 1 mg/kg, check ACT again in 3-5 min
      e.   If ACT still < 450, give 2u FFP or antithrombin III
      f.   Redose heparin 1 mg/kg 2h after loading dose and repeat q1h thereafter
      g.   For HIT pt, consider argatroban or hirudin
2.   Amicar (aminocaproic acid, EACA)
      a.   Plasminogen inhibitor
      b.   Normally given shortly after heparin
      c.   10 mg bolus followed by 2 mg/h infusion
3.   Aprotinin
      a.   Plasmin inhibitor and preserve plt function
      b.   Risk of anaphylactic reaction requiring testing dose
      c.   Only for high risk bleeding pt
      d.   Monitored by kaolin-ACT

Monitor During Bypass
1.   BP
      a.   Maintained 50-80 mmHg
      b.   Differential of hypotension (<30 mmHg)
         -   Preload: venous cannula malposition
         -   Pump: insufficient flow rate or pump malfunction

- Afterload: aortic dissection
   c. Treatment of HTN (> 100 mmHg)
- Reduce flow rate
- Add isoflurane
- Add vasodilator such as nitroprusside
2. Flow: ~ 2.5 L/min/m^2
3. ABG
   a. α-stat management
- Use uncorrected gas tension
- Does not require adding CO_2 into system
- Preserve autoregulation of cerebral blood flow
- Commonly used in adult cases
   b. pH-stat management
- Use corrected gas tension as "normal" CO_2 tension 40 mmHg and pH 7.4
- May need to add CO_2 into system
- Used in pedi cases
- Blood seems to be alkalotic during hypothermia 2/2 low CO_2 tension
4. Hct: Keep > 18% (20-25%), UOP > 1 ml/kg/h
5. CVP and PA should be ~ 0

Termination of CPB
1. General guidelines for separation from CPB
   a. Core body temp > 37 °C
   b. Stable rhythm
   c. HR ~ 80
   d. BP ~ 80
   e. Adequate ventilation with 100% O_2
   f. Reasonable lab results
2. Weaning off CPB
   a. Defibrillate (5-10 J) if heart fibrillates
   b. Lidocaine 100 mg if defibrillation fails
   c. Pacing HR ~ 80
   d. Ca^{++} 15 min after release of cross-clamp in divided dose
   e. Hand vent with 100% O_2 with short inspiration to remove air from pulm circulation
3. Protamine reversal of heparin
   a. Binds heparin
   b. 1 mg of protamine for 1 mg of heparin, 250 mg bolus followed by gtt
   c. Check ACT 3-5 min later
   d. Side effects
- Hypotension
- Pulm HTN
- Myocardial depression
- Allergic reaction in pt taking NPH
4. Post-CPB bleeding
   a. Differential

- Poor surgical control
- Inadequate protamine reversal
- Heparin rebound
  - Protamine to peripheral component or heparin to central component
- Coag deficiency
- Thrombocytopenia or plt dysfunction
- Hypothermia

  b. Treatment
  - FFP
  - Plt transfusion (keep plt >100K)
  - DDAVP

5. Medications
   a. Dobutamine - ↑ CO, minimal change in BP
   b. Dopamine - ↑ both CO and BP
   c. Epinephrine - more potent, ↑ both CO and BP
   d. Milrinone - ↑ CO, ↓ BP and PVR
   e. Norepinephrine - ↓ CO, ↑ BP
   f. Nitric oxide, TNG and prostaglandin E1 - ↓ PVR
6. Intraaortic balloon pump
   a. Inflated just after closure of aortic valve
   b. Deflated just before LV ejection
   c. ↑ Coronary blood flow without increase in cardiac work

Surgery of Descending or Abdominal Aorta

Dissection classification
1. DeBakey classification
   a. Type I – Originates in ascending aorta, propagates at least to the aortic arch and often beyond it distally
   b. Type II – Originates in and is confined to the ascending aorta
   c. Type III – Originates in descending aorta
2. Stanford classification
   a. Type A – Originates in ascending aorta
   b. Type B – Originates in descending aorta

General anesthesia concerns
1. A-line on right radial because left subclavian artery clamping might be necessary
2. HTN after aorta clamping
   a. May precipitate acute CHF and/or MI
   b. May exacerbate AR
   c. Less dramatic if clamp is more distal
   d. Nitroprusside may be necessary
3. Hypotension after release aorta clamping has the greatest hemodynamic instability
   a. Physiology

- ↓ Afterload
- Flush of acid metabolites and K^+

    b. Treatment
- ↓ Depth of anesthesia
- IV fluid
- Vasopressor
- Might need Ca^{++}

4. Spinal cord ischemia and paraplegia
    a. General Information
- Mostly in thoracic aorta surgery
- Anterior spinal artery syndrome
      • Motor and pain/temperature sensory defects
      • Vibration and proprioception remains
- Adamkiewicz artery mostly at left T9-T12
    b. Prevention
- Shunt
- CSF drainage
- CSF cooling
- Steroid
- Mannitol
- SSEP & MEP monitor

5. Renal failure
    a. Significantly reduces renal blood flow
    b. Prevented with mannitol and fenoldopam prior cross-clamp

Transplanted Heart

1. Denervated, therefore absence of vagal influence
2. Normal or enhanced response to circulating catecholamine
3. High resting HR
4. CO is preload dependent
5. Two sets of P waves
6. Indirect vasopressors are less effective than direct-acting agents
7. Isoproterenol or diluted epinephrine should be readily available to increase HR
8. Silent MI
9. Immunosuppressive meds (for most transplantation patients)
    a. Corticosteroids
    b. Cyclosporine
    c. Tacrolimus

Pulmonary HTN (Anesthesia Concerns)

1. Avoid N_2O
2. Avoid hypercarbia

3. Avoid high airway pressure
4. Avoid acidosis
5. High FiO$_2$
6. Milrinone
7. TNG
8. Nitric Oxide
9. Prostaglandin E1

Chapter 6 Neuro

Neurological Monitors

EEG
1. BIS
   a. 40 – 60 as general anesthesia
   b. Keep volatile > 0.7 MAC is as effective as BIS (NEJM 2008)
   c. Consider BIS for TIVA
2. EEG
   a. Activate: N_2O, ketamine, low dose anesthetics
   b. Depress: high dose anesthetics except N_2O and ketamine
      - Isoflurane is the only volatile to produce flat EEG

Evoked potentials
1. SSEP: monitor dorsal column
2. MEP: monitor ventral spinal cord, esp. in aorta surgery
3. Auditory evoked potentials: monitor brain stem function in posterior fossa surgery
4. Volatiles ↓ amplitude and ↑ latency
5. IV anesthetics and N_2O have much less effect
6. Etomidate and ketamine ↑ SSEP amplitude

50% decrease
Amplitud
60% increase
latency

① Optimize Spinal Perfusion
↑HTN, ↑Hte, ↑FiO₂, ↓ETCO₂

③ Rule Out deep Anesthesia
③ Rule Out excessive distraction
→ If persistent: wake up test.

Intracranial Hypertension

Definition
1. ICP > 15 mmHg,
2. Life threatening if ICP > 40 mmHg
3. Normal ICP < 10 mmHg

Clinical Presentation
1. History: HA, N/V, MS change
2. Physical exam: Papilledema, Cushing response (HTN with bradycardia)
3. Specific test: CT – midline shift >0.5 cm

Physiology
1. CPP = MAP – ICP (or CVP, whichever is higher)
2. Normal CBF 50 ml/100g/min (750 ml/min, 20% CO)
   a. CBF autoregulated if MAP 60-160 mmHg
   b. CBF increases with ↑ CO_2 (2 ml/100g/min/mmHg $PaCO_2$ change)
   c. CBF remains unchanged to PaO_2 till PaO_2<50 mmHg
   d. CBF change ~ 5% every 1 °C temperature change
      - CMR ↓ 50% for every ↓ 10 °C
      - EGG flat at 20 °C
3. Cerebral O_2 consumption 50 ml/min (20% of total O_2 consumption of 250 ml/min)

4. Intracranial compliance
   a. Poor compliance: ↑ ICP > 4 mmHg with 1 ml injection
5. Major compensatory mechanism
   a. CSF from brain to spine (initial)
   b. Decrease CSF production
   c. Increase CSF absorption
   d. Decrease cerebral blood volume

Treatment
1. Mechanical
   a. Rev T burg
   b. CSF drainage
   c. Burr hole
2. Hyperventilation (to $PaCO_2$ ~ 30 mmHg)
3. Medication
   a. Decadron (esp. vasogenic edema, such as tumor)
   b. Mannitol (~ 1 g/kg)
      - Wait till dura is opened in intracranial bleeding
      - Serum osmolarity up to 310 mOsm (normal 280-290)
      - Max effect in 10 min
      - Last 3-4 h
   c. Lasix
   d. 3% saline
   e. Thiopental
4. Fluid restriction
5. Do Not Use LUMBAR DRAIN (IS FOR BRAIN RELAXATION)

ICP monitor
1. Intraventricular catheter with ventriculostomy (gold standard)
2. Subdural/subarachnoid bolt
   a. Transducers of ICP and A-line at ear

Effects of anesthetics
1. CMR: all decrease except ketamine
2. CBF:
   a. Inhalational – ↑
      - Autoregulation is impaired by volatile anesthetics
      - CBF-$PaCO_2$ response remains with volatile
      - Steal phenomenon
   b. IV drugs – ↓ (except ketamine)
      - Thiopental – reverse steal phenomenon
3. ICP:
   a. Inhalational – ↑ (isoflurane and N_2O minimal)
   b. IV drugs – ↓ (except ketamine)
4. Sux: mild increase of CBF and ICP, which can be prevented by NDMR priming
5. Narcotics: little effect on CBF, CMR, or ICP
6. Intubation in lightly anesthetized pt greatly ↑ ICP
7. Routine neuro use:

a. Isoflurane for regular neuro cases
b. TIVA if dura is tight

Anesthesia concerns
1. Slow controlled induction
2. Avoid hyper or hypotension
3. Sux is OK, although it increases ICP
4. Sufficient relaxant to prevent cough unless MEP
5. Mild hyperventilation
6. Avoid PEEP if possible
7. NS (rather than LR)

Head Trauma

Intracranial bleeding
1. Epidural hematoma
    a. Lens like appearance on CT
    b. Tearing of middle meningeal artery
    c. Lucid interval (1/3 unconscious at time of injury, 1/3 lucid interval, 1/3 never unconscious
2. Subdural hematoma
    a. Crescent appearance on CT
    b. Most common type of intracranial hematoma
    c. Laceration of bridging vein between dura and draining sinuses
    d. Immediate comatose in severe acute subdural hematoma
3. Subarachnoid hematoma
    a. Aneurysm rupture is the most common cause
    b. Vast majority at circle of Willis
    c. 10% acute mortality
4. Intracerebral
    a. AVM
5. Skull fracture

Glasgow Coma Scale (GCS)
1. Eye opening (4 points)
2. Verbal response (5 points)
3. Motor response (6 points)
GCS 8 or less defined as coma, intubation is required;
GCS 9-12 is moderate

What are your concerns (system)?
1. Neurological
    a. Increased ICP that causes decreased CBF
    b. Cervical spinal cord injury
        - C-spine can be clinically cleared if patient has none of the following:
            • Neck pain

- Severe distracting pain
- Neurological signs or symptoms
- Intoxication
- Loss of consciousness
  - CT scan to rule out
    - Negative predictive value of 98.9 for ligament injury and nearly 100% for unstable c-spine injury

2. Respiratory
   a. Airway obstruction
   b. Aspiration
   c. Chest injury (PTX)
   d. Neurogenic pulmonary edema (due to sympathetic stimulation)
3. Cardiac
   a. ECG changes similar to MI
   b. HTN
   c. Hypotension indicates other additional injuries
      - Control of hypotension and bleeding is more important that imaging studies or neurosurgical treatment
4. GI
   a. Esophageal, gastric, or duodenal ulcers
   b. GI bleeding
   c. Prophylactic antacid therapy
5. Hem
   a. DIC
6. Endo
   a. Diabetes insipidus
   b. SIADH
      - Treat with demeclocycline, an ADH antagonist

Ruptured Intracranial Aneurysm

Symptoms
1. Sudden onset of HA
2. Symptoms of increased ICP
3. Loss of consciousness
4. Meningeal signs
5. The most common cause of subarachnoid hemorrhage
6. 10% acute mortality

Complications
1. Rerupture
   a. Peak in 1st wk
   b. 60% mortality
   c. #1 reason for early surgery is to prevent rebleeding (< 3d)
2. Vasospasm
   a. Caused by blood clot around cerebral vessels

      b.   4-14 days after rupture
      c.   Presentation: new neurological defects, delayed neurological deterioration
      d.   Diagnosis: transcranial Doppler (increase velocity) and angiogram
      e.   Prevention: nimodipine, early surgery
      f.   HHH therapy: Hypertension, Hypervolemia, Hemodilution
3. Hydrocephalus
4. Seizure

EKG changes
1. Common with SAH (50-100%)
2. Do not correlate with MI
3. 3 possibilities for Q waves
      a.   MI
      b.   SAH induced MI
      c.   No MI

Anesthesia induction
1. Maintain stability: prevent both HTN (for rerupture) and hypotension (for hypo-perfusion)
2. Mannitol after dura is opened

Issues with Posterior Fossa Surgery

Anesthesia concerns
1. Brainstem injury (respiratory and circular centers)
2. Venous air embolism
3. Pneumocephalus
      a.   No N_2O
4. Obstructive hydrocephalus

Venous Air Embolism

Detection
1. TEE: most sensitive
2. Precordial Doppler (right parasternal 2nd intercostal space): 0.25 ml detectable
3. PAC: increase pulm pressure
4. Decrease $ETCO_2$
5. Increase ETN_2

Treatment
1. Notify surgeon: Surgical field protection – NS flooding and bone wax
2. Central line aspiration
3. Left lateral T burg (release air lock from RV outflow track)
4. Stop N_2O

5. iv fluid to ↑ CVP
6. Vasopressors
7. Jugular vein compression (to ↓ air entry)
   a. Complications:
      - ↓ CBF
      - Cerebral edema
      - Carotid artery compression
      - Bradycardia
8. No PEEP (may induce paradoxical embolism)

Placement of multi-orifice central line
1. Tip should at superior vena cava-RA junction (2 cm below SA node)
2. Place with intravascular EKG at biphasic p wave
3. Confirm with CXR

Acromegaly (Pituitary Tumor of Growth Hormone)

What are your concerns (system)?
1. Respiratory
   a. Large nose, lips, and mandible: difficult to mask
   b. Large tongue, tonsils, epiglottis: difficult to intubate
   c. OSAS?
   d. Awake FOI first choice, large blade, small tube, emergency airway ready
2. Cardiac
   a. HTN
   b. Acromegalic cardiomyopathy
3. Neuro
   a. CN II (Lateral visual field defects; optic chiasm compression)
   b. CN III, IV, V defects
4. Endo
   a. Hyperglycemia

Problems for transsphenoidal pituitary tumor resection (tumor <10 mm)
1. Intramucosal epinephrine absorption
2. Blood and tissue accumulation in pharynx and stomach
3. Internal carotid artery and cavernous sinus injury
4. CN injury
5. Post-op diabetes insipidus
   a. Polydipsia, polyuria
   b. Urinary osmolarity < plasma osmolarity

Anesthesia for transsphenoidal
1. Steroid (hydrocortisone 100 mg) and antibiotics before induction
2. No N_2O (pneumocephalus)
3. Intensive muscle relaxant (microscopic surgery)
4. Lumbar intrathecal cath (maybe) to drain CSF for better surgical exposure

5. Post-op treatment of diabetes insipidus (DDAVP)

Pituitary function
1. Anterior pituitary hormones: prolactin, ACTH, GH, TSH, LH, FSH
2. Posterior pituitary hormones: ADH (released when serum osmolarity ~290), oxytocin

CEA (Carotid Endarterectomy)

Pre-op eval
1. Cardiac eval for CAD
2. OK to stop coumadin for a few days

Neurological monitor
1. Awake pt is the best monitor
2. EEG is the gold standard for GA pt
3. Transcranial Doppler
4. Stump pressure: shunt if <50 mmHg
    a. Collateral perfusion:
        -   Contralateral internal carotid
        -   Basilar
        -   Vertebral
5. Xenon washout

GA vs. RA
1. Both GA and RA are OK
2. GA is preferred because of secure airway and $PaCO_2$ control
    a. Avoid complications of deep and superficial cervical block
    b. Need monitor for cerebral ischemia

Intraop hemodynamic control
1. Although HTN may increase perfusion, BP is normally kept within pre-op range b/o possible cerebral edema
2. Bradycardia can develop during carotid sinus manipulation
3. Hypotension following carotid unclamping

Stroke pt
1. Postpone elective surgery after a complete stroke for at least 6 weeks
2. Avoid Sux
3. Avoid twitch monitor on paralyzed side because of NDMR resistance

Postop stroke
1. Overall risk is low
2. Higher in cardiovascular surgery
3. Highest in open heart surgery for valvular disease and operation on thoracic aorta

Spinal Cord

Blood supply
1. Anterior spinal artery (from vertebral artery) – supplies anterior 2/3 of spinal cord
   a. Anterior cord syndrome: loss of motor function, pain and temperature sensation
2. Posterior spinal artery – supplies posterior 1/3
3. Radicular arteries
   a. Adamkiewicz (radicularis magna): most common at left T9-11

Spinal cord injury
1. Pre-op considerations
   a. Injury above C3-5 (diaphragmatic innervation) requires vent support
   b. Injury above T1-4 reduce cardiac and pulmonary sympathetic innervation (acute)
   c. Injury above T6 can develop autonomic hyperreflexia (chronic)
   d. Most common sites of transaction are C5-6 and T12-L1
   e. Acute transaction causes spinal shock for weeks (loss of sensation, flaccid paralysis, loss of reflex below injury)
2. Anesthetic considerations
   a. Acute transection
      - Neck injury clearance
      - Awake FOI or in-line stabilization with RSI/cricoid pressure if neck is not cleared
      - Sux is OK for first 24 h
      - A-line is indicated, CVP and PAC are helpful
      - High dose of steroid in 1st 24 h
   b. Chronic transection
      - Autonomic hyperreflexia
        • HTN below level of lesion
        • Vasodilation above the level of lesion
        • Regional anesthesia and deep general anesthesia to prevent
        • Nitroprusside, nitroglycerin, and hydralazine should be available
      - Hyperkalemia
        • NMBAs is preferred

Visual Loss with Spinal Surgery (ASA Advisory 2006)

Causes for visual loss with spinal surgery
1. Posterior ischemic optic neuropathy
2. Anterior ischemic optic neuropathy
3. Central retinal artery occlusion

Risk factors
1. Spine surgery (prone position) (< 0.2% of spine surgeries)

2. Prolonged procedure
3. Substantial blood loss

ASA advisory 2006

> 6.5h
> 45% EBL

1. Inform high risk pt −
2. Staged spine procedures in high risk pt
3. High-risk pt should be positioned in a neutral position and to keep head level with or higher than heart   (looking forward)
4. No specific transfusion threshold to reduce risk of periop visual loss , Avoid Hypotension

ECT

Physiology
1. Initial parasympathetic discharge
    a. Marked bradycardia
    b. Consider premed with glycopyrrolate
2. Sustained sympathetic discharge
    a. HTN and tachycardia

Contraindication
1. MI < 3 mon
2. Stroke < 1 mon
3. Increased ICP
4. Intracranial mass

Anesthesia considerations
1. Methohexital is the most common induction agent
2. Low dose propofol (1 mg/kg) can be used
3. Benzo raises seizure threshold and decrease duration
4. Sux is most often used muscle relaxant
5. Mask ventilation

Seizure

Causes
1. Structural brain lesion – head trauma, tumor, stroke
2. Metabolic abnormality – uremia, liver failure, drug withdrawal
3. Idiopathic

Types
1. General – loss of consciousness
2. Partial – no loss of consciousness

Management of seizure

1. ABC
2. Medication
    a. Thiopental iv 50-100 mg
    b. Versed iv 1-5 mg

Anesthesia considerations
1. Preop
    a. Continue anti seizure medication till surgery
    b. Barbiturates increase hepatic microsomal enzyme
2. Intraop
    a. Medications should be avoided:
        - Methohexital, ketamine, etomidate, meperidine,
    b. Phenytoin and carbamazepine ↑ requirement of nondepolarizing relaxant
3. Postop
    a. Resume anti seizure med ASAP
    b. Delayed arousal may be due to postictal state

Anesthesia Concerns for Other Neurological Diseases

Parkinson's disease
1. Continue PD medication
2. Avoid reglan and droperidol
3. Can have hyper or hypotension after induction if taking levodopa
4. Can develop NMS if withdrawal PD meds

Multiple sclerosis
1. Postpone elective surgery during relapse
2. Avoid hyperthermia (increase temperature makes symptoms worse)
3. Avoid spinal anesthesia
4. Epidural anesthesia is OK

MAO inhibitor
1. Chess and wine (tyramine) causes HTN
2. Meperidine and MAOI can cause fever and seizure
3. Avoid indirect vasopressor
4. Increase response to sympathetic stimuli

TCAs
1. Avoid indirect vasopressor
2. Increase response to sympathetic stimuli

Lithium
1. Prolong the duration of muscle relaxant
2. Can cause wide QRS complex
3. Can cause diabetes insipidus
4. Can cause hypothyroidism

Neuromuscular Diseases

Myasthenia Gravis
1. Pathophysiology
   a. Antibody to postsynaptic acetylcholine receptor leading to less receptors
   b. Muscle weakness with repeated activity
   c. Associated with thymoma or thymic hyperplasia
   d. Clinical improvement after thymectomy
   e. Treat with cholinesterase inhibitor (pyridostigmine), steroid, plasmapheresis
   f. Cholinergic crisis
      - Excessive cholinesterase inhibitor
      - Differentiate from myasthenic crisis by edrophonium test
        • Get better → myasthenic crisis
        • Get worse → cholinergic crisis
2. Anesthesia considerations
   a. Preop
      - Continue cholinesterase inhibitor to prevent periop weakness
      - Aspiration prophylaxis for pt with bulbar or respiratory involvement
      - No premed
   b. Intraop
      - Regional anesthesia preferred
      - Awake FOI for pt with bulbar or respiratory involvement
      - Deep volatile anesthesia alone may provide sufficient relaxation for intubation
      - More sensitive to nondepolarizing NMBA (small dose if use)
      - Response to sux is unpredictable (either resistant or phase II block)
   c. Postop
      - Post-op vent support might be necessary, esp. thymectomy pt

Lambert-Eaton
1. Pathophysiology
   a. Antibody to Ca^{++} channels to ↓ Ach release
   b. Associated with small cell carcinoma of lung
   c. Muscle weakness improves with repeated effort
   d. Treat with guanidine and diaminopyridine, which stimulate Ach release
2. Anesthesia considerations
   a. Regional anesthesia preferred
   b. Very sensitive to both depolarizing and non-depolarizing NMBAs
   c. Deep volatile anesthesia alone may provide sufficient relaxation for intubation

Duchenne Muscular Dystrophy
1. Pathophysiology
   a. The most common and most severe form of muscular dystrophy
   b. X-linked recessive
   c. Diagnosed by muscle biopsy

    d. Can cause severe scoliosis
    e. Respiratory muscle degeneration causes respiratory failure and recurrent pulmonary infection
    f. Cardiac muscle degeneration causes heart failure and arrhythmia

2. Anesthesia considerations
    a. Regional anesthesia preferred
    b. Avoid sux b/o possible association with MH
    c. Might be sensitive to nondepolarizing NMBA
    d. Marked respiratory and cardiac depression with volatile

Myotonic Dystrophy

1. Pathophysiology
    a. Slowing of relaxation after muscle contraction
    b. Respiratory involvement leads to decreased vital capacity
    c. Cardiac involvement leads to arrhythmia
    d. GI involvement leads to aspiration

2. Anesthesia concerns
    a. Very sensitive to sedatives, inhalational and iv anesthetics, and opioids
    b. Premed can cause sudden and prolonged apnea
    c. Sux is relatively contraindicated because it causes intense myotonic contractions and possible MH
    d. The response to nondepolarizing NMBA is normal
    e. The reversal of nondepolarizing NMBA can cause induce myotonic contraction
    f. Postop shivering can induce myotonic contraction
    g. Prolonged postop pulmonary complications

Chapter 7 GI/Liver

Cirrhosis

What are your concerns (Systems)?
1. Respiratory
    a. Aspiration: GI bleeding
    b. Oxygenation: ↓ FRC, hypoxemia from right-to-left shunt (systemic and intrapulmonary)
    c. Ventilation: pleural effusion
2. Cardiovascular
    a. ↑ Preload
    b. High cardiac output (hyperdynamic circulation)
    c. Cirrhotic cardiomyopathy
    d. ↓ Afterload (low SVR)
3. Neuro
    a. Encephalopathy
        - Aggravated by:
            • GI bleeding
            • Protein intake
            • Infection
            • Vomiting /diuresis
        - Treat with lactulose /neomycin
4. GI
    a. Portal HTN (> 10 mmHg)
        - Esophageal varices
        - Hemorrhoids
        - GI bleeding
            • Treatment
                a. Vasopressin
                b. Propranolol
                c. Balloon tamponade
                d. Endoscopic sclerosis
                e. TIP (transjugular intrahepatic portosystemic shunt)
    b. Ascites / spontaneous bacterial peritonitis
    c. Hepatic dysfunction
    d. Jaundice
5. Hematology
    a. Coagulopathy
    b. Vit K deficiency
    c. Thrombocytopenia (congestive splenomegaly)
    d. Anemia
6. Renal
    a. Hepatorenal syndrome
    b. Na and water retention (Treatment: water and sodium restriction)

7. Endo/metabolic
    a. Hyponatremia
    b. Hypokalemia
    c. Hypomagnesemia
    d. Hypoglycemia
    e. Hypoalbuminemia

Lab Tests
1. Enzymatic
    a. ↑ ALT/AST (cellular dysfunction)
    b. ↑ Alkaline phosphatase (cholestasis)
2. Synthetic (nearly all proteins)
    a. ↓ Albumin (nl > 3.5, half life 3 wks)
        - ABCD: increase free Barbiturates, Coumadin, Diazepam
    b. ↓ Clotting factors (except factor VIII and von Willebrand factor)
        - PT (nl 11-14s) for factors V, VII, and X
        - Factor VII has shortest half life (6 h)
        - Extrinsic pathway is more important in vivo
    c. ↓ Pseudocholinesterase (half life 14 days) (Sux, mivacurium, ester LA)
3. Bilirubin ↑
    a. Indirect (unconjugated)
        - ↑ Production: hemolysis
        - ↓ Conjugation decrease liver disease
    b. Direct (conjugated)
        - Biliary obstruction

Anesthesia considerations
1. Pre-op
    a. FFP?
    b. Vit K?
        - Works in biliary obstruction, not as much in hepatocellular damage
        - Need 24 h to have full effect
2. Intraop
    a. RSI with cricoid pressure (if N/V, GI bleed, Abd distension)
    b. Muscle relaxant
        - Initial dose: high (increased volume of distribution)
        - Maintenance dose: low (slow metabolism)
        - Hepatic elimination: pancuronium, rocuronium, vecuronium
    c. Maintain with isoflurane (volatile with least effect on hepatic blood flow)
    d. Colloid (albumin) preferred
    e. Citrate toxicity
3. Extubation
    a. Fully awake

Child's Classification
1. Albumin
2. Ascites

3. Bilirubin
4. Encephalopathy
5. Nutrition

Jaundice

What do you think (differential)?
1. Prehepatic (unconjugated, indirect bilirubin) (Most likely the cause in postop)
    a. Hematoma absorption
    b. RBC breakdown after transfusion
2. Hepatic
    a. Hepatic ischemia
    b. Hepatic congestion
    c. Hepatitis
    d. Medication (halothane hepatitis)
3. Posthepatic

Opioids and Sphincter of Oddi Spasms
    Fentanyl > morphine > meperidine

Alcoholism

What are your concerns (systems)?
1. Respiratory
    a. Risk of aspiration
2. Cardiovascular
    a. Alcoholic cardiomyopathy: CHF, arrhythmia
3. Neuro
    a. MAC ($\downarrow$ acutely, $\uparrow$ chronically)
    b. DT
    c. Wernicke-Korsakoff syn.: thiamine deficiency
    d. Neuropathy: B12/folate deficiency
4. GI
    a. Esophagitis, gastritis
    b. Pancreatitis
5. Liver
    a. Fatty liver
    b. Acute alcoholic hepatitis (AST > ALT)
    c. Cirrhosis

Bowel Obstruction

What are your concerns?

1. Respiratory
    a. Risk of aspiration
    b. ↓ FRC from abd distension
2. Cardiac
    a. Hypovolemia from fluid sequestration
    b. Septic shock
3. Electrolytes
    a. Volume depletion alkalosis
    b. Metabolic acidosis from hypoperfusion
    c. Respiratory acidosis

Chapter 8 Hematology

Blood Type

1. Type & Screen takes 5 min
2. Type & Cross takes 45 min (indirect Coombs test)
3. Emergency: O (-)
4. FFP and cryo can be given regardless of Rh status
5. ABO compatible plt is desirable but not necessary

Transfusion (ASA Guidelines 2006)

RBC transfusion
1. Hb < 6 g/dl should be transfused (Hb 6 g/dl can be tolerated by young healthy patient)
2. Hb > 10 g/dl should not be transfused
3. Should consider the potential of ongoing bleeding
    a. 1 u PRBC ↑ Hb ~1 g/dl

Platelets transfusion
1. plt < 50 in presence of excessive bleeding indicates platelets transfusion
2. plt > 100 rarely indicates plt transfusion
3. plt dysfunction, even with enough plt account
    a. 1 u plt ↑ plt count ~ 10K

FFP transfusion indications
1. Urgent reversal of coumadin therapy
2. Correction of known factor deficiencies
3. Excessive microvascular bleeding with INR > 2.0 or PTT greater than 2 times normal or INR and PTT cannot be obtained in a timely fashion
4. Heparin resistance (antithrombin III deficiency) in pt requiring heparin
5. Not indicated for augmentation of plasma volume or albumin concentration
6. To achieve minimum of 30% factor concentration: 10 ml/kg
7. Urgent reversal of coumadin: 5 ml/kg

Cryoprecipitate transfusion indication
1. Pt with congenital fibrinogen deficiency
2. von Willebrand disease pt if specific concentrates not available
3. Fibrinogen < 100 mg/dl with excessive microvascular bleeding
4. To correct excessive microvascular bleeding in massively transfused patients when fibrinogen cannot be measured in a timely fashion

Drugs to treat excessive microvascular bleeding (coagulopathy)
1. Desmopressin (DDAVP)
2. Topical hemostasis

    a. Fibrin gel
    b. Thrombin gel

Adverse effects of transfusion
1. Bacterial contamination
    a. Leading cause of death from blood transfusion
    b. Most common in plt product
    c. Suspect sepsis if pt develops fever within 6 h after plt transfusion
2. TRALI
    a. Can appear 1-2 h after transfusion and peak at 6 h
    b. Recover in 4 days
    c. Critical care support
    d. One of the most common causes of transfusion related death
3. Infectious disease
4. Transfusion reaction
    a. Monitor peak airway pressure
    b. Monitor urine output and color

Transfusion Hemolytic Reaction

1. Signs and Symptoms
    a. Hypotension
    b. Tachycardia
    c. Hemoglobinuria /ARF
    d. Wheezing
    e. Fever
    f. DIC
2. Test
    a. Direct Comb test
    b. Plasma free Hb
3. Management
    a. Stop transfusion
    b. Recheck blood product
    c. Keep U/O: Foley, iv fluid, ± mannitol
    d. Hemodynamic support
    e. Lab: CBC, coag

Massive Transfusion

Definition
1. 1-2 times of total blood volume
2. ~ 10-20 units

What are your concerns?

1. Side effects of transfusion
2. Bleeding
    a. Dilutional thrombocytopenia
    b. Dilutional factor defects
3. Electrolyte
    a. Acid-base balance
        - Post-op metabolic alkalosis
        - Metabolic acidosis (uncommon)
    b. Citrate toxicity /↓ Ca^{++}
        - In fast transfusion (> 1u/5 min)
        - In hepatic dysfunction or hypothermic pt
        - Need Ca^{++} infusion
    c. Potassium ~ ↑ 4 mEq/u

Other Transfusion Techniques

1. Cell-saver
    a. Contraindicated in sepsis and cancer
    b. Only when blood loss > 1L
2. Autologous transfusion
    a. Not risk free: contamination, labeling error, allergic reaction
    b. Requires Hb > 11 g/dl
3. Isovolemic hemodilution

Synthetic Colloids

1. Hextend (hetastarch)
    a. Anaphylactic reaction is rare
    b. Coag and plt dysfunction when > 1L
2. Dextran
    a. Anaphylactoid and anaphylactic reaction can happen
        - Dextran 1 prior to Dextran 40 or 70 to prevent
    b. Antiplatelet effect
    c. Dextran 40 improves microcirculation

DIC (Disseminated Intravascular Coagulation)

Pathophysiology
1. Widespread deposition of fibrin in the microcirculation
2. Consumption of coag factors
3. Fibrinolysis, thrombocytopenia, and hemolytic anemia
4. Diffuse bleeding
5. Thromboembolic event may happen

Causes
1. Sepsis
2. Shock
3. Placenta abruption
4. MH
5. TURP
6. Transfusion hemolytic reaction

Lab
1. ↑ PT, PTT
2. ↓ Fibrinogen

Treatment
1. Treat underlying causes
2. Transfuse FFP, plt, cryoprecipitate
3. Amicar is contraindicated

Sickle Cell Disease

Pathophysiology
1. Hb β chain glutamate (HbA) to valine (HbS) at sixth position
2. ~ 10% African American has trait (heterozygous HbSA), ~ 1% African American has disease (homozygous HbSS)
3. HbSA pt is asymptomatic with possible renal concentrating abnormality
4. Less O_2 affinity (HbS P_{50} = 31 mmHg, HbA P_{50} = 27 mmHg)
5. HbS polymerizes and precipitates with low O_2 (factors that moves Hb curve to right)
   a. Hypoxia
   b. Dehydration
   c. Acidosis
   d. 2,3-DPG increase
   e. Temperature increase
6. HbSS sickles when O_2 sat < 80% (normal venous sat), HbSA sickles if O_2 sat < 40%
7. HbSS red cell has 1/10 survival time (12 vs. 120 days)

What are your concerns?
1. Pulmonary
   a. Pulmonary infarct
   b. Recent lung infection
2. Cardiac
   a. MI
   b. CHF
   c. Cor pulmonale
3. Neuro
   a. Stroke
   b. Seizure

73

4. Hem
    a. Anemia
    b. Spleen infarct /functional asplenia
    c. Splenic sequestration
    d. Recurrent infections
5. GI
    a. Hepatic infarct
    b. Cholecystitis
6. Renal
    a. Hematuria
    b. Renal failure
    c. Impaired renal concentration ability

Major complications
1. Vaso occlusive crises
    a. Most painful crises are due to microinfarcts in various tissues
    b. Acute abd, chest, back, joint pain
    c. Can result in splenic, cerebral, pulmonary, hepatic, and myocardial infarctions
    d. Functional splenectomy by adolescence
2. Splenic sequestration crisis
    a. Caused by occlusion of spleen venous drainage
    b. Causes hypovolemic shock
    c. Occurs in infants and young child
    d. Treated by emergency splenectomy
3. Aplastic crisis
    a. Profound anemia (Hb 2-3 g/dl)
    b. Occurs in children ages 4-10
    c. Infection and folate deficiency play a major role

Precipitation factors of sickle cell crisis (same as factors for precipitation except hypothermia)
1. Hypoxia
2. Dehydration
3. Acidosis
4. Hypothermia
5. Infection

Treatment of sickle cell crisis
1. O_2
2. Hydration
3. Treat underlying condition

Diagnosis
1. Suspect for sickle cell if African American with h/o jaundice or joint/bone/abd pain
2. Sickledex screen test
3. Hb electrophoresis to confirm

Anesthesia considerations

1. Pre-op
    a. Consider exchange transfusion, goal:
        - Hb ~ 10 g/dl
        - HbAA 50%
    b. Hydration, infection control
2. Intra-op
    a. $FiO_2 > 50\%$
    b. Avoid dehydration, hypotension, acidosis, hypo/hyperthermia
    c. Avoid tourniquets
3. Post-op
    a. Most periop death occur in post-op period
    b. Hypoxia and pulmonary complications are major risk factors

von Willebrand Disease

1. von Willebrand factor facilitates the function of plt and factor VIII
2. The most common inherited bleeding disorder
3. Increase bleeding time
4. Treat with cryoprecipitate and factor VIII concentrate
5. DDAVP for type I and IIA, but causes thrombocytopenia in type IIB

Porphyria

Pathophysiology
1. Enzyme deficiencies in heme biosynthetic pathway
2. Results in metabolic intermediates accumulated

Signs and Symptoms
1. Abdominal pain
2. Vomiting
3. Neurological symptoms
4. Photosensitivity

Drugs are unsafe for porphyria
1. Barbiturates
2. Reglan
3. ACE inhibitors
4. Calcium channel blockers

Drugs are potentially unsafe for porphyria
1. Etomidate
2. Ketamine
3. Hydralazine
4. Clonidine

Chapter 9 Electrolyte

Potassium

EKG changes
1. PR prolongation in both hypo- and hyperkalemia
2. QRS complex: widened in hyper
3. ST depression in both hypo and hyper
4. T wave: peaked in hyper, flattened in hypo
5. U wave: in hypo

Acute treatment for hyperkalemia
1. Ca^{++}
2. Hyperventilation /bicarb
3. Insulin/glucose (1 u insulin/50 g of glucose)
4. β2 agonist (albuterol) /epinephrine – activates Na^+/K^+ pump, release insulin
5. Lasix
6. Dialysis
7. Kayexalate

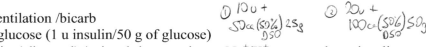

Hypokalemia (Anesthesia concerns)
1. Cutoff for elective surgery: K^+ 3.0 if no EKG change or symptoms, except on digoxin
2. Small dose of muscle relaxant
3. Avoid hyperventilation
4. 20 mEq K^+ supplementation increase K^+ level ~0.1 mEq/L

Calcium

Regulation
1. PTH (increase)
2. Vit D (increase)
3. Calcitonin (decrease)

Hypercalcemia
1. Most common causes are malignant and hyperparathyroidism
   a. Check PTH to differentiate
2. Treat with in fluid and lasix

Hypocalcemia
1. Signs and Symptoms
   a. Muscle spasm
   b. Arrhythmia
   c. Decreased heart contractility
2. 1 gram of $CaCl_2$ has 3 times of Ca^{++} compared to 1 gram of calcium gluconate

Anion Gap

Definition
1. $[Na^+] - [Cl^-] - [HCO_3^-]$
2. Normal range 7-14 mEq/L

Metabolic Acidosis (Primary ↓ of $[HCO_3^-]$)

Anion Gap acidosis
1. Endogenous
    a. DKA
    b. Lactate
    c. Uremia
2. Exogenous ~~Renal Failure~~
    ~~Rhabdo~~
    ~~Starvation~~ ~~Toxins~~

Dilutional Acidosis expanders
Glycase
SIADH

Normal Anion Gap acidosis (hyperchloremic)
1. GI loss
    a. Diarrhea
    b. Fistula
    c. (Ureterosigmoidostomy)
2. Renal loss
    a. ACEI (Hypoaldosteronism)
    b. Diamox (acetazolamide, carbonic anhydrase inhibitor)
3. Increased intake

Respiratory Acidosis and Alkalosis (Normal pH 7.35-7.45)

*   Acute respiratory acidosis – For each 10 mmHg ↑ $PaCO_2$ above 40 mmHg, $[HCO_3^-]$ ↑ 1 mEq/L from 24 mEq/L, pH ↓ 0.1

*   Chronic respiratory acidosis – For each 10 mmHg ↑ $PaCO_2$ above 40 mmHg, $[HCO_3^-]$ ↑ 4 mEq/L from 24 mEq/L

*   Acute respiratory alkalosis – For each 10 mmHg ↓ $PaCO_2$ below 40 mmHg, $[HCO_3^-]$ ↓ 2 mEq/L from 24 mEq/L

*   Chronic respiratory alkalosis – For each 10 mmHg ↓ $PaCO_2$ below 40 mmHg, $[HCO_3^-]$ ↓ 4 mEq/L from 24 mEq/L

Chapter 10 Renal

Renal Anesthesia Concerns

1. Methoxyflurane and enflurane cause fluoride toxicity
2. Sevoflurane produces compound A
3. Autoregulation with MAP 80-180 mmHg; GRF=0 if MAP 40 mmHg
4. Aminoglycoside and contrast can cause renal damage
5. GRF < 25 ml/min is renal failure
6. Indigo carmine can cause HTN or hypotension

Uremia

1. Respiratory
   a. Aspiration: ↓ gastric emptying, N/V
   b. O_2: hypoxia 2/2 pulm edema
   c. Vent: ↑
2. Cardiovascular
   a. Preload: ↑
   b. Pump: CHF, arrhythmia, pericarditis
   c. Afterload: HTN
3. Neuro
   a. Encephalopathy
   b. Autonomic neuropathy
4. Hem
   a. Anemia
   b. Plt dysfunction
5. Metabolic
   a. Metabolic acidosis
   b. Hyperkalemia

[handwritten margin note: Uremia with CHF — Metabolic Acidosis ↓HCO_3 w Resp Alkalosis ↓$PaCO_2$]

TURP Syndrome

What are your concerns (systems)? (hyponatremia and hypervolemia)
1. Pulmonary
   a. Pulmonary edema
   b. Dyspnea
2. Cardiovascular
   a. Preload: ↑
      - Hypervolemia: 20 cc/min absorption
      - Lithotomy position
   b. Pump:
      - EKG change (Na^+ >105 mEq/L): widened QRS, ST elevation

- VT/Vfib ($Na^+ > 100$ mEq/L)
- CHF

    c. Afterload: hypotension
3. Neuro ($Na^+ < 120$ mEq/L acutely)
    a. HA, restless, confusion
    b. Seizure
4. Hematology:
    a. Hemolysis
5. Electrolytes
    a. Hyponatremia
    b. Hypoosmolarity
    c. Hyperglycinemia

Risk Factor
1. Duration of surgery
2. Height of irrigation fluid

Treatment (correct Na^+ to > 125 mEq/L)
1. Stop surgery
2. NS (Na^+ 154 mEq/L)
3. Fluid restriction
4. Lasix
5. 3% NS ($Na^+ > 500$ mEq/L) if $Na^+ < 120$ mEq/L , stop till Na^+ 120-130 mEq/L
6. Slow Na^+ correction (< 1.5 mEq/L/h) to avoid central pontine myelinolysis (quadriplegia)
7. Best monitor for hyponatremia is mental status: try TURP with regional

Concerns for TURP surgery
1. TURP syndrome
2. Bladder perforation
    a. Signaled by poor fluid return
    b. Abd pain, nausea, diaphoresis, shoulder pain
    c. Bradycardia (vagal), HTN, hypotension
3. Sepsis
4. Hemorrhage
    a. Can be caused by release of fibrinolytic enzymes
    b. Can be treated with Amicar (plasminogen inhibitor)
5. DIC
6. Hypothermia
7. Regional anesthesia (T10 level) preferred to catch early signs of TURP syndrome and bladder perforation

Lasix

1. Increase renal secretion of Na^+, Cl^-, K^+, H^+
2. Acts at ascending loop of Henle

Chapter 11 Endo

Diabetes Mellitus

What do you think (system)?

1. Respiratory
    a. Airway: Stiff-joint syndrome – TMJ, cervical spine
    b. Aspiration: Gastroparesis
2. Cardiovascular
    a. CAD
    b. Peripheral vascular disease
    c. Autonomic neuropathy (50% DM pt with HTN)
    d. Painless MI, HTN, orthostatic hypotension, resting tachy, reduced HR response to atropine and β blocker
3. Neurological
    a. Autonomic neuropathy
    b. Peripheral neuropathy
4. Endo (three life threatening acute complications)
    a. DKA
    b. Nonketotic hyperosmolar coma
    c. Hypoglycemia
5. Renal
6. Nephropathy

Change in Functional Status + Important than Functional Status

Classification

- Type I – Absolute insulin deficiency (immune-mediated or idiopathic)
- Type II – Adult onset (insulin resistance/relative deficiency)
- Type III – Other genetic defects
- Type IV – Gestational

Life threatening emergencies

1. DAK
    a. In type I DM
    b. Infection is the most common cause
    c. Sign/Symptom: tachypnea, hypotension, tachycardia, mental status change, N/V, abd pain
    d. Treatment: IV fluid, insulin, potassium
        - Several L of NS (rather than LR) is required
        - Reduce glucose 10%/h
        - W5D once glucose reaches 250 mg/dl
2. Nonketotic hyperosmolar coma
    a. In type II DM
    b. Osmolarity can be as high as 360
    c. Na^+ ↓ 1.6 mEq/L for every 100 mg ↑ of glucose
    d. Signs: mental status change

    e. Treatment: IV fluid, insulin, potassium
3. Hypoglycemia
    a. Signs: diaphoresis, tachycardia

Adverse effect of intraop hyperglycemia
1. DKA
2. Nonketotic hyperosmolar coma
3. Worse neurological outcome following stroke
4. Worse outcome after cardiac surgery and acute MI
5. Associated with infection and poor wound healing

Anesthesia management
1. Preop
    a. Half of morning dose of insulin
    b. Hold AM dose of PO hypoglycemic med
    c. Hold metformin for 24 h
2. Intraop
    a. Monitor glucose q1h in type I pt, q2h in type II pt
    b. Keep glucose 120-150 mg/dl
    c. Hyperglycemia treatment (> 180 mg/dl)
      - Bolus: 1 u regular insulin ↓ glucose 25-30 mg/dl
      - Infusion: units per hour = glucose level / 150
    d. Hypoglycemia treatment (< 100 mg/dl)
      - 15 cc of D50 ↑ glucose 30 mg/dl
    e. Risk of anaphylaxis
      - Protamine in pt taking NPH or PZI (long acting)

Obesity (BMI > 30)

What are your concerns (system)?
1. Respiratory
    a. Airway:
      - Difficult airway
      - OSAS
    b. Aspiration
      - ↓ Gastric emptying
      - ↑ Gastric acid
    c. Oxygenation: hypoxia
      - ↑ Closing capacity
      - ↓ FRC
      - ↑ V/Q mismatch
    d. Ventilation: obesity-hypoventilation syndrome (Pickwickian syndrome)
      - Hypercarbia
      - Cyanosis-induced polycythemia
      - Right heart failure
      - Somnolence

Monitoring: A-line — NIBP non reliable.

2. Cardiac
    a. CAD
    b. HTN
    c. Pulm HTN from hypoxia
3. Endo
    a. DM
    b. Other: hypothyroidism, Cushing's

Pheochromocytoma

General information
1. Symptoms
    a. Paroxysmal HA, palpitation, diaphoresis, HTN
    b. Hypovolemia
    c. Hyperglycemia ($\alpha 1$ activity inhibits insulin release)
    d. Catecholamine induced cardiomyopathy
    e. Part of MEN type II
    f. 10% malignant, 10% extra adrenal, 10% bilateral
2. Diagnosis
    a. Serum and urinary catecholamines and their metabolites (E, NE, VMA)

Anesthesia concerns
1. Preop
    a. $\alpha 1$ antagonist phenoxybenzamine or prazosin PO
    b. β blocker only after α blocker
    c. Volume replacement
2. Intraop
    a. Phentolamine (slow onset), nitroprusside, esmolol
    b. Avoid ketamine, anticholinergics, pancuronium, histamine release meds, sux
    c. Intubate only after pt is deeply anesthetized
3. Postop
    a. Might develop hypotension from hypovolemia and/or catecholamine tolerance
    b. Postop HTN may indicate residue tumor

Hyperthyroidism

Pathophysiology
1. TRH – TGH – T4/T3
2. T3 is more potent and is converted from T4 peripherally
3. Graves' disease is #1 cause of hyperthyroidism
4. Iodine inhibits release and synthesis of T4/T3

Treatment
1. Inhibit synthesis – propylthiouracil

2. Inhibit release – iodide
3. Control adrenergic over activity – propranolol (also inhibits release)
4. Cell damage – radioactive iodine
5. Surgery

Anesthesia concerns
1. Preop
   a. Postpone elective surgery until pt is euthyroid, including subtotal thyroidectomy
   b. Esmolol infusion for emergent surgery
   c. Watch for possible airway compression and volume depletion
2. Intraop
   a. Avoid ketamine and pancuronium
   b. Be careful about muscle relaxant for possible myasthenia gravis
   c. Intubate only when pt is deeply anesthetized
   d. Pt can be hypovolemic
   e. Avoid indirect adrenergic agents.
   f. No change in MAC
3. Postop
   a. Thyroid storm
      - The most serious postop thread to hyperthyroid pt
      - Can occur intraop
      - Clinical features
        • High fever, tachycardia, hypotension, MS change, death
        • No muscle rigidity or metabolic/respiratory acidosis
      - Precipitating factors
        • Surgery, stress, infection, iodine withdrawal
      - Treatment
        • Hydration, cooling, esmolol infusion, propylthiouracil (NG tube), iodine, steroid
   b. Airway issues after thyroid surgery
      - Recurrent laryngeal nerve damage
      - Hematoma
      - Tracheomalacia
      - Laryngeal stridor /laryngospasm – hypocalcemia from hypoparathyroidism
      - PTX

Carcinoid Syndrome

1. Secretion of vasoactive substance
2. Flushing, bronchospasm, diarrhea, swings of BP
3. Associated with right-side heart disease
4. Somatostatin to reduce the secretion
5. Urine Metabolite for Diagnosis

Chapter 12 OB

Physiological Changes

1. Respiratory
   a. Airway
      - ↑ Risk of upper airway obstruction from capillary engorgement of mucosa
      - Small ET tube
      - Big breasts
   b. Aspiration
      - ↑ Gastric volume
      - ↑ Gastric acid
      - ↓ Gastroesophageal sphincter
   c. Oxygenation
      - FRC ↓ 20%
      - Rapid oxygen desaturation during apnea
      - O_2 consumption ↑ 20%
      - PaO_2 ↑ 10%
   d. Ventilation
      - Vm ↑ 50%
      - Vt ↑ 40%
      - RR ↑ 15%
      - $PaCO_2$ ↓ to 28-32
      - $[HCO_3^-]$ ↓ to 21
      - ABG at term: 7.44/30/100
      - Can have resp. alkalosis during labor that decreases uterine blood flow
   e. Hb
      - ↓ to 11 g/dl
      - P_{50} ↑ to 30 mmHg
      - 2,3 DPG ↑
2. Cardiovascular
   a. Preload
      - Blood volume ↑ 35% (↑ ~ 1L at term)
      - Plasma volume ↑ 45% (Hb ↓ to 11)
      - IVC and aorta compression (after 28 wk)
        • Left uterus displacement
        • Shunt from paravertebral veins to azygous vein
      - Venous stasis /phlebitis
   b. Pump
      - CO
        • ↑ 40% at term
        • ↑ Another 40% during labor
        • ↑ Another 40% immediately after delivery (highest)
        • Return to nl in 2 wks

- Stroke volume ↑ 30%
- HR ↑ 20%
- Mild systolic murmur
  c. Afterload
- SBP ↓ 5%
- DBP (SVR) ↓ 15%
- Pulmonary resistance ↓ 30%
3. Neuro
   a. GA
- MAC ↓ 40% from ↑ progesterone level
- Rapid inhalation induction from low FRC and high MV
   b. LA
- Dose requirement ↓ 30%
- Epidural venous plexus distension
  - ↑ Epidural pressure
  - ↓ Epidural space
  - ↓ CSF volume
4. Hem
   a. Hb 11
   b. Iron and folate acid anemia
   c. Hypercoagulable state: ↑ fibrinogen and all factors (except XI)
- PE is the #1 cause of pregnancy related mortality
   d. Thrombocytopenia in preeclampsia
5. Hepatic
   a. ↓ Pseudocholinesterase (Sux, mivacurium, ester LA)
   b. ↓ Albumin
   c. ↑ Alkaline phosphatase from placenta secretion
6. Renal
   a. GFR ↑ 50%
   b. Mild glycouria and proteinuria (< 300 mg/d)
   c. [HCO_3^-] compensated to 21
7. Endo
   a. Hyperglycemia
   b. ↑ Total T3 & T4, normal free T3/T4
   c. ↓ Serum Ca, normal ionized Ca^{++}
8. Musculoskeletal
   Prone to back pain from ligament relaxation

Anesthesia Concerns of Ob Epidural

1. 1st stage level: T10-L1
2. 2nd stage level: T10-S4
3. C/S and tubal ligation level: T4
4. Both ephedrine and phenylephrine are OK to treat hypotension
5. Ketamine 10-15 mg as adjuvant for patchy RA

Pregnancy-Induced HTN

Definition
1. PIH
   a. SBP > 140 mmHg or DBP > 90 mmHg
   b. Or 30/15 mmHg above baseline
2. Preeclampsia
   a. HTN
   b. Proteinuria > 500 mg/d
   c. Edema
   d. Occur after 20 wk of pregnancy
   e. Resolve 2 days after delivery (can happen postpartum)
3. Severe preeclampsia
   a. BP > 160/110 mmHg
   b. Proteinuria > 5 g/d
   c. Edema
      - Pulmonary edema leads to CHF
      - Upper airway edema leads to obstruction
      - Cerebral edema leads to HA and visual disturbance
   d. Oliguria (< 500 ml/d) (from severe hypovolemia)
   e. Hepatic tenderness
   f. HELLP syndrome
      - <u>H</u>emolysis
      - <u>E</u>levated <u>L</u>iver enzyme
      - <u>L</u>ow <u>P</u>latelet
4. Eclampsia
      Preeclampsia with seizure

What are your concerns (system)?
1. Respiratory
   a. Airway: upper airway edema
   b. Lung: pulmonary edema
2. Cardiovascular
   a. Preload: intravascular hypovolemia
   b. Pump: CHF (pulm edema)
   c. Afterload: HTN, Increased SVR
3. Neuro
   a. Seizure
   b. Stroke
   c. HA
   d. Visual disturbance
4. Hem
   a. Thrombocytopenia
   b. plt 70K is OK for epidural
   c. DIC
5. GI/Hepatic
   a. Elevated liver enzymes

    b. Hepatic tenderness
6. Renal
    a. Proteinuria
    b. Oliguria
    c. Decreased GRF

Etiology
1. Not clearly known
2. Placental ischemia caused by immunologic reaction
3. Subsequent release of rennin, angiotensin, and aldosterone
4. Primarily affects first pregnancy
5. Incidence increase with rapid uterus enlargement: diabetes, multiple gestations
6. Maternal death due to pulm edema, stroke, and hepatic necrosis or rupture

Treatment
1. Best rest
2. Magnesium
    a. 4 g loading dose over 20 min
    b. 2 g/h infusion
    c. 6-8 mg/dl therapeutic level (nl ~2 mg/dl)
        -   10 mg/dl – deep tendon reflex loss
        -   15 mg/dl – resp. depression
        -   20 mg/dl – cardiac arrest
        -   Calcium gluconate antagonizes most of the effects of hypermagnesia
3. Anti-HTN medication
    a. Labetalol 5-10 mg iv (esmolol has adverse fetal effect)
    b. Hydralazine 5 mg iv
    c. TNG or nitroprusside (cyanide toxicity if > 10 mcg/kg/min) for severe cases
4. Delivery of fetus and placenta (definitive treatment)
5. Treatment of eclampsia
    a. ABC: intubation
    b. Control seizure: thiopental 50-100 mg – Mg Bolus 4g/20min
        Phenytoin
        lorazepam
        thiopental

Anesthesia considerations
1. A-line for severe HTN
2. If epidural is considered
    a. Check plt and coag, plt > 70K is OK for epidural – Dr. Li motion 75-100K, >100K is ofut
    b. Check volume status
3. Reduced dose of relaxant if pt is on Mg^{++}
4. Small dose of vasopressor for hypotension

Bleeding

Partum Hemorrhage
1. Placenta abruption
    a. Separation of placenta from uterine wall after 20 wk

    b.   painful vaginal bleeding with uterine contraction and tenderness
    c.   Diagnosed by US
    d.   DIC can develop
    e.   Severe abruption is life threatening and needs emergent C/S under GA
2.   Placenta previa
    a.   Placenta completely or partially cover or close to internal cervical os
    b.   Painless vaginal bleeding
    c.   Diagnosed by US
    d.   C/S. Low-lying placenta might try vaginal delivery
    e.   Bleeding can continue after delivery from poor contraction of implantation site
    f.   Risk factors: large placenta, advance maternal age, h/o C/S or uterine myotomy
    g.   h/o placenta previa and C/S increase risk of placenta accreta, increta, and percreta
3.   Uterine rupture
    a.   Abrupt onset of severe continuous abd pain & hypotension
    b.   Fetal distress, loss of uterine tone

Postpartum Hemorrhage (severe bleeding is #1 obstetric morbidity)
1.   Uterine atony
    a.   Risk factor
     - Uterine overdistension – multiple gestation, large fetus
     - Retained placenta
    b.   Treatment
     - Uterine massage
     - Oxytocin
       • Half life 5 min
       • 40 u/L iv
       • Vasodilation causes hypotension and tachycardia
     - Methergine
       • 0.2 mg im
       • Vasoconstriction causes THN and coronary spasm
     - Hemabate
       • 0.25 mg im, Q15-90 min prn, max 2 mg
       • Vasoconstriction causes HTN
       • Avoid in asthma pt
       • Hypoxia – ↑ V/Q mismatch
       • N/V, diarrhea
     - Ligation of internal iliac artery
     - Hysterectomy
2.   Retained placenta
    a.   GA to relax uterus
    b.   Nitroglycerine may be used as an alternative
3.   Uterine inversion   *50-100mcg bolus – Fast-titrate to effect*
4.   Laceration   *– Treat hypotension with Neo/Ephe.*

Preterm Labor

1. Delivery 24-37 wks
2. Surfactant is not sufficient before 35 wks
3. Betamethasone for 48 h
4. β2 agonist and Mg^{++} to delay labor

Fetal Monitoring

How do you monitor fetus?
1. Baseline HR: 110-160
2. Baseline variability
   a. Decreased baseline variability is a sign of fetal asphyxia
   b. Meds can decrease baseline variability: opioids, benzo, Mg, atropine
3. Accelerations (> 15 beats/min for > 15 s)
   a. Absence of baseline variability and acceleration is "nonreassuring"
4. Decelerations
   a. Early decelerations: fetal head compression
   b. Late decelerations: uteroplacental insufficiency
   c. Variable decelerations: umbilical cord compression
5. Scalp pH
   a. pH < 7.2 is associated with fetal depression

Neonatal Resuscitation

Apgar Score (total of 10)

Score	0	1	2
HR	0	<100	>100
Respiration	none	irregular	crying
Muscle Tone	none	some	full
Reflex	none	grimace	cry
Color	blue	pink/blue	pink

1. 1 min score correlates with survival
2. 5 min score correlates with neurological outcome

Immediate care
1. Apgar score 5-7: face mask
2. Apgar score 3-4: hand vent
3. Apgar score 0-2: intubate

Mask ventilation indication
1. Apnea
2. HR < 100
3. Gasping respiration

4. Persistent central cyanosis with 100% O_2
    a. Initial breaths with peak pressure 40 cmH$_2$O
    b. Subsequent breaths with peak pressure 30 cmH$_2$O

Intubation indication
1. HR < 60
2. HR 60-80 for 30 s after 100% O_2 mask ventilation
3. Ineffective ventilation
4. Prolonged mask ventilation
5. Need to give medication

Cardiac compression indication
1. HR < 60
2. HR 60-80 for 30 s after 100% O_2 mask ventilation
    a. Chest compression 120/min
    b. Stop when HR > 80
3. Epinephrine (10-30 mcg/kg) iv or ETT if asystole or HR < 60 despite compression
4. Check pulse at femoral or brachial

Ob GA Routine

1. LUD
2. IV access
3. Monitor
4. Pre-O$_2$
5. Prep & drape
6. RSI and cricoid pressure
7. Intubation with small ETT
8. Volatile/N$_2$O/O$_2$ (sevo if preferred because it has less effect on ventilation) (<1MAC required)
9. NDMR prn
10. Avoid hyperventilation (hypocapnia reduces uterine/placental blood flow)
11. D/C volatile after delivery, keep N$_2$O (to prevent Uterine Atony)
12. Oxytocin gtt after delivery

  - Mortality rate for GA is more than 10 times higher than that of RA
  - Life of mother takes priority over life of fetus

Postpartum Tubal Ligation

Anesthesia concerns
1. Usually within 48 h of vaginal delivery
2. Still at risk of aspiration
3. If epidural is used for delivery, test epidural before to OR. T4 level, as C/S
4. If GA, RSI, relatively low concentration of volatile

5.   Avoid breast feeding 12-24 h after GA

Postpartum Headache

What do you think (differential)?
1.   PDPH
2.   Primary headache
      a.   Migraine
      b.   Tension headache
      c.   Cluster headache
3.   Withdraw headache: caffeine, pain killer
4.   Secondary HA
      a.   Bleeding: SAH/SDH
      b.   HTN
      c.   Infection: meningitis, sinusitis

Anesthesia During Pregnancy

Teratogenic effect
1. 3rd to 8th week is the most critical period
2.   Past concerns in N_2O (inhibits myelin and DNA synthesis) and benzodiazepines (palate malformation) are not justified

Timing of surgery
1.   Elective surgery should be postponed till 6 wks after delivery
2.   End of 2nd trimester (20-24 wks) are good window for urgent surgery

Anesthesia issues
1.   Regional is preferred
2.   Fetal monitor if more than 24 wks
3.   β2 agonist to abort preterm labor

Fluid Neonates
Maintenance with Glucose 4 cc/kg/h
Replacement 6 cc 6-8
Blood Loss 1:1 Albumin RBC

Chapter 13 Pedi

General Concerns

Physiological features
1. Respiratory
   a. Airway
      - Large head and tongue
      - Narrow nasal passage
      - Anterior and cephalad larynx (C4 rather than C6 in adult)
      - Long epiglottis
      - Cricoid cartilage is the narrowest point (up to 5 yrs)
      - Short trachea and neck
   b. Aspiration
      - High incidence of reflex
   c. Oxygen
      - High O_2 consumption (6 cc/kg/min vs adult 3 cc/kg/min)
      - Low FRC
      - Quickly develops hypoxia during apnea
   d. Ventilation
      - Vt per kg is the same as adult
      - High RR
      - Less efficient ventilation from weak costal and diaphragm muscle
      - Less respiratory drive to hypoxia or hypercarbia
   e. Hb
      - HbF
2. Cardiovascular
   a. Pre-load
      - Hallmark of hypovolemia is hypotension without tachycardia (< 1 yr)
   b. Pump
      - Fixed stroke volume
      - CO is rate dependent
      - Most common cause of neonatal bradycardia is hypoxemia
   c. Afterload
      - Blunted response to exogenous catecholamines
3. Neuro
   a. MAC is higher in infants than in neonate and adult
   b. Rapid inhalational induction from high alveolar ventilation and low FRC
   c. Require lager dose of propofol and thiopental
   d. Muscle Relaxants
      - Faster onset
      - Require less amount (except sux, cis, and mivacurium)
      - Higher dose of succinylcholine (2-3 mg/kg)
      - Profound bradycardia and arrest can occur after 1st sux (Pre-treat Atropine)

Routine
Controversial use
♂ < 8yo ↑
-Replace ROC (1mg/kg)
double intubating dose

0.02 mg/kg

4. Renal
   a. Low GFR

   b. Low concentration ability
5. Hem
   a. Hb: 75% HbF at birth, 100% HbA at 6 mon
6. Metabolism
   a. Greater heat loss can cause hypothermia
   b. Brown fat metabolism is the major source of heat production
   c. Low glycogen storage can predispose hypoglycemia

Pedi Anesthesia Numbers

Average body weight: $(Age \times 2) + 9$
ETT ID: $Age/4 + 4$
ETT length: $Age/2 + 12$

HR
 Neonate: 140 (fetal 110-160)
 1 yr: 120
 3 yr: 100
 12 yr: 80
BP
 Neonate: 65/40
 1 yr: 95/65
 3 yr: 100/70
 12 yr: 110/60
RR
 Neonate: 40
 1 yr: 30
 3 yr: 25
 12 yr: 20
Blood Volume
 Premature neonate: 100 ml/kg
 Full term neonate: 90 ml/kg
 Infant: 80 ml/kg
 Adult: 70 ml/kg
Hb
 Neonate: 17 g/dl
 3 mon: 10 g/dl
 6 mon: 12 g/dl

Upper Respiratory Infection

1. ↑Airway reactivity for 4 weeks
2. ↑ Risk for respiratory related adverse events such as laryngospasm, post-extubation croup, bronchospasm

3. Postpone elective case
    a. Discuss with surgical team
    b. Cancel for 2 wks for mild URI
    c. Cancel for 4 wks for wheezing and productive cough
    d. Practical approach: given the frequency of URI and difficulty of surgical scheduling, it may more practical to allow surgery to proceed, esp. for myringotomy tubes, T&A, and cleft palate repair, which might actually resolve URI with surgery
    e. Definitely cancel the case if pt has fever or pneumonia

Hypothermia

What are your concerns (systems)?
1. Pulmonary
    a. Respiratory depression
    b. Hb: left shift of Hb curve
2. Cardiovascular
    a. Pump: arrhythmia, decrease contractility
    b. Afterload: ↑ SVR
3. Neuro
    a. Delayed awakening from anesthesia
    b. ↓ MAC
    c. Neuroprotective to global ischemia
4. Hem
    a. plt dysfunction
    b. Coagulopathy
    c. ↑ Infection
5. GI/Hepatic
    a. ↓ Drug metabolism
    b. Potential citrate toxicity after transfusion
6. Renal
    a. ARF

Risk factors for pedi pt
1. Thin skin
2. Low fat content
3. High surface relative to weight
4. No shivering

Malignant Hyperthermia

Pathophysiology
1. Abnormal calcium channel receptors (ryanodine receptor) on sarcoplasmic reticulum
2. Uncontrolled Ca^{++} release from sarcoplasmic reticulum

3. Dantrolene binds ryanodine receptor and inhibits Ca^{++} release
4. Diagnosed by muscle biopsy with halothane-caffeine contraction test
   a. 90% specificity, ~100% sensitivity
   b. Only a few centers worldwide do it
   c. Voluntary
   d. Not in little child (because the amount of muscle is too significant)
5. 50% pt have previous uneventful exposure to triggering agents
6. 50% masseter muscle spasm (trismus) pt develops MH
7. Associated with musculoskeletal diseases (such as Duchenne's muscular dystrophy)
8. 1:15,000 in pedi, can occur in adult
9. Genes on several chromosomes are linked to MH

Signs of MH
1. Hypermetabolism
   a. ↑ CO_2 production (early sign and sensitive indicator)
   b. ↑ O_2 consumption
   c. Low mixed venous oxygen tension
   d. Metabolic acidosis (mixed with respiratory acidosis)
2. ↑ Sympathetic activity
   a. Tachycardia (early sign)
   b. Arrhythmia (VF, the most common cause of death, can develop as quick as 15 min)
   c. Initial HTN, followed by hypotension
3. Muscle damage
   a. Generalized rigidity (not consistently present)
   b. Dark urine (Myoglobinuria)
   c. Myoglobinemia
   d. Hyperkalemia
   e. Elevated creatine kinase
4. Hyperthermia (late sign, can rise $1\,^{\circ}C$ every 5 min)
5. DIC

Differential
1. MH
2. Neuroleptic malignant syndrome
   a. Functional dopamine deficiency
   b. Causes
      - Antidopaminergic treatment
        • Neuroleptic meds
        • Reglan
        • Droperidol
      - Levodopa withdrawal in Parkinson's pt
   c. NDMR can reverse rigidity (but not in MH)
   d. Dantrolene and levodopa can also reverse rigidity
3. Thyroid storm
   a. Generally develops in post-op (6-24 h after surgery) but can occur intraop
   b. Pts with undiagnosed or poorly controlled hyperthyroidism

      c.   Presents as high fever, hypotension, tachycardia, MS change
      d.   Not associated with muscle rigidity, elevated CK, or metabolic/respiratory acidosis
      e.   Low K^+ is common (unlike hyperkalemia in MH)
      f.   Treatment: hydration, cooling, β blockers, propylthiouracil, sodium iodide, cortisol
4. Serotonin syndrome
      a.   High fever, HTN or hypotension, resp. arrest, coma
      b.   Causes
         -   MAOI and meperidine
         -   MAOI and SSRIs
         -   Illicit drugs: cocaine, PCP, LSD
5. Sepsis
6. Transfusion reaction

MH Protocol
1. Call for help
2. Discontinue causing agents and Breathing
      a.   Discontinue volatile and Sux
      b.   Change anesthesia tubing and soda lime
3. 100% O_2 with hyperventilation
4. Dantrolene
      a.   2.5 mg/kg q 5 min, max 4 doses (10 mg/kg)
      b.   20 mg mix with 60 ml water
      c.   Subsequent 1 mg/kg q6h for 24-48h (half life 6h)
      d.   Given through a central line because it can cause phlebitis
      e.   May result in generalized weakness that causes respiratory insufficiency
      f.   Can be used in neuroleptic malignant syndrome
5. Monitor: UO, A-line, CVP
6. Lab: Chem 7, ABG, CBC, Coag (DIC)
7. Targeted Treatments
      a.   Hyperthermia
      b.   Acidosis
      c.   Hyperkalemia
      d.   Renal
      e.   Hemodynamic
8. Call 1-800-MH-HYPER

Prematurity

Retinopathy of prematurity
1. Infants younger than 44 weeks postconception are at risk
2. Fibrovascular proliferation in retina
3. Associated with high O_2 tension
4. Oxygen level fluctuation is more harmful than high O_2 tension
5. Normal PaO_2 60-80 mmHg in neonate (normal fetal PaO_2 40 mmHg)

Post-op apnea
1. Preterm infants younger than ~~50~~ 44 weeks postconceptional are at risk
2. Elective surgery should be deferred until preterm infant reaches ~~50~~ 44 wk postconception
3. For surgery in preterm infants less than ~~50~~ 44 wks postconceptional, post-op monitor 24 h

Necrotizing Enterocolitis
1. Intestinal ischemia and bacterial overgrowth
2. Septic shock, hypovolemia, DIC

Pyloric Stenosis

Pathophysiology
1. Symptoms occur most commonly at 2-6 wks of age
2. Volume depleted metabolic alkalosis
3. Low Na^+, Cl^-, and K^+

Anesthesia Considerations
1. Preop
   a. Postpone surgery till fluid and electrolytes are corrected
   b. Hydration with NS with K^+ supplementation
2. Intraop
   a. Gastric tube suction with pt in supine, lateral, and prone positions
   b. Awake intubation or RSI
3. Postop
   a. High risk of post-op respiratory depression 2/2 persistent metabolic alkalosis

Tracheoesophageal Fistula

1. Type IIIB is most common
2. Other congenital abnormalities (cardiac) are common
3. G-tube suction and avoid positive pressure ventilation before intubation
4. Awake intubation without muscle relaxants
5. May need 100% O_2 despite risk of retinopathy of prematurity

Gastric distention with positive pressure
↳ *Qx Gastrostomy*

Congenital Diaphragmatic Hernia

1. Pulmonary hypoplasia and pulm HTN are common, pt may need ECMO and NO
2. G-tube suction and avoid positive pressure ventilation before intubation
3. Awake intubation
4. No N_2O because of pulm HTN, hypoxia and air expansion in the bowel
5. Be aware of PTX

Down Syndrome

What are your concerns (systems)?
1. Respiratory
   a. Airway
      - Irregular dentition
      - Small jaw
      - Large tongue
      - Atlantoaxial subluxation
      - Subglottic stenosis
   b. Lower airway: tracheoesophageal fistula
   c. Lung: chronic pneumonia
2. Cardiovascular
   a. VSD
   b. Endocardial cushion defects
3. Neuro: seizure

Chapter 14 Other Topics

Laparoscopic Surgery

Physiological effect of pneumoperitoneum
1. Respiratory
    a. Airway
        - ↑ Risk of aspiration
        - Trachea shift upward → ETT to right main stem (esp. with T-burg)
    b. Oxygen
        - ↓ FRC
        - ↑ V/Q mismatch and shunt
    c. Vent
        - ↑ Inspiration pressure
        - ↑ Vm because of CO_2 absorption
2. Cardiac
    a. Preload
        - Unchanged or slightly increased with moderated insufflation pressure
        - ↓ If insufflation pressure >25 cmH_2O
    b. Pump
        - Tachycardia and arrhythmia 2/2 hypercarbia
    c. Afterload
        - HTN if hypercarbia
3. Renal
    a. Oliguria from venous and kidney compression

Anesthesia considerations
1. GETA is preferred
    a. Prevent aspiration
    b. Vent control to prevent hypercarbia
    c. Provide sufficient inspiration pressure

Complications
1. CO_2 embolism
    a. Treatment
        - Immediate release pneumoperitoneum
        - Stop N_2O
        - Central line for aspiration
        - Left lateral T-burg
2. Vagal stimulation
    a. Causes
        - Trocar insertion
        - Peritoneum insufflation
        - Manipulation of viscera
3. PONV

4. Pneumomediastinum and PTX

Rheumatoid Arthritis

What are your concerns (systems)?
1. Respiratory
    a. Airway
        - Atlantoaxial subluxation
            • Compressing spinal cord and compromising vertebral blood blow
            • Pre-op flexion/extension lateral cervical X-ray if pt takes steroid or methotrexate
            • If atlantoaxial instability > 5mm, need inline stabilization or awake FIO
            • If atlantoaxial instability > 9mm, need surgical fusion
        - TMJ: limited mouth opening
        - Cricoarytenoid joint
            • Small glottic opening: hoarseness, stridor
            • Smaller ETT
    b. Lung
        - Pulmonary fibrosis
        - Pleural effusion
        - Pulmonary nodules
2. Cardiac
    a. Cardiac nodules with conduction abnormality
    b. Pericardial effusion & thickening
    c. Valvular disease
3. Neuro: nerve root compression from rheumatoid nodules
4. Hem
    a. Anemia
    b. Plt dysfunction from NASIDs
5. Endo: adrenal insufficiency form steroid
6. Musculoskeletal: symmetric arthritis

Scoliosis

What are your concerns (systems)?
1. Pulmonary
    a. Oxygenation
        - ↑ V/Q mismatch
        - Chronic hypoxia
    b. Ventilation
        - Restrictive lung disease
        - May need post-op ventilation

2. Cardiovascular
   a. Mitral prolapse
   b. Pulm HTN from chronic hypoxia: EKG – RVH, right axis deviation, RBBB
3. Musculoskeletal: scoliosis caused by muscular dystrophy has high risk of MH and abnormal response to sux.

Specific Concerns in Orthopedic Surgery

Fat embolism
1. Following long-bone or pelvic fracture
2. Trial of dyspnea, confusion, and petechiae (petechiae is diagnostic clue)
3. Prevented by early stabilization
4. Supportive treatment

DVT
1. Most common in hip surgery and TKR
2. Neuraxial anesthesia may reduce DVT
3. Prophylactic anticoagulation
4. Pneumatic leg compression
5. Early ambulation

Bone cement implantation syndrome
1. Signs
   a. Hypotension, arrhythmia, hypoxia (increase shunt), pulm HTN
2. Anesthesia concerns
   a. Increase FiO_2 before cementing
   b. Keep euvolemia
   c. PAC for bilateral THR and TKR

Tourniquets
1. Tourniquet pain
   a. Presented as gradual increase of BP ~ 1 h after inflation in GA pt
   b. Cuff deflation immediately relieves pain and HTN
2. Tourniquet release hypotension
3. Can cause PE
4. Prolonged (> 2 h) tourniquet may cause nerve and muscle injuries

Anaphylactic Reaction

Clinical Manifestation
1. Respiratory
   a. Laryngeal edema
   b. Bronchospasm
   c. Pulmonary edema

2. Cardiac
    a. Tachy
    b. Arrhythmia
    c. Hypotension
3. Skin
    a. Urticaria
    b. Itchiness
    c. Facial edema

Differential from Anaphylactoid
1. Clinically indistinguishable
    a. Equally life-threatening
    b. Same treatment
2. Check tryptase for anaphylactic reaction
3. IgE causes anaphylactic reaction, requires prior exposure to antigen
4. Muscle relaxant is the most common cause of anaphylactic reaction, latex allergy 2nd
    a. Pt with spina bifida, spinal cord injury, GU tract malformation have high incidence of latex allergy
5. IgA deficiency pt receiving IgA blood transfusion can cause anaphylactic reaction

Treatment
1. Stop causing drug
2. ABC (intubation)
3. 100% O_2
4. IV fluid
5. Epinephrine (10 to 500 mcg)
6. Benadryl
7. Ranitidine
8. Steroid (hydrocortisone up to 200mg)

Burn

Systems
1. Respiratory
    a. Upper airway obstruction: from edema (early intubation)
    b. Oxygenation:
        - Chemical pneumonitis (can be initially symptom free)
        - Pulmonary edema /ARDS
        - ↓ Compliance from chest wall injury
    c. Ventilation: ↑ Vm because of high metabolism
    d. Hb – CO toxicity
        - Falsely high reading with regular oximeter
        - COHb can be detected by laboratory CO-oximeter
        - Hb dissociation curve to left
        - Treat with 100% O_2, hyperbaric O_2 can be considered
2. Cardiovascular

a. Preload: hypovolemia initially
   - 4 ml/kg/% Parkland formula or LR first 24h
   - 50% of total fluid in first 8h
   b. Pump: hyperdynamic 24h later
3. Electrolytes
   a. Hyperkalemia in acute phase
   b. Hypokalemia in chronic phase
4. Renal
   a. Keep U/O > 1 ml/kg/h
   b. ARF
5. GI: Curling's ulcer & GI bleeding

Geriatrics

What are your concerns (system)?
1. Respiratory
   a. Common Pulm diseases: COPD
   b. Aspiration: ↓ gastric emptying time
   c. Oxygenation: ↑ closing capacity & V/Q mismatch, ↓ PaO_2
   d. Ventilation: Blunted response to hypoxia and hypercarbia
2. Cardiac
   a. Common Cardiac diseases: CAD, HTN, CHF
   b. Pump: ↓ CO, ↓ response to β blocker
   c. Afterload: ↑ SVR, ↑ BP drop after induction
3. Neuro
   a. ↓ Requirement for both general and local anesthetics
   b. Likely to have postop cognitive dysfunction
4. Renal
   a. ↓ GFR
   b. Creatinine stable
5. Hepatic: prone to drug overdose from reduced liver blood flow and reduced protein binding

Ophthalmic Surgeries

Intraocular Pressure
1. Inhalation and iv anesthetics (except ketamine) decrease intraocular pressure
2. Sux and ketamine increase intraocular pressure
3. Intubate only after deeply anesthetized to prevent coughing

Oculocardiac Reflex
1. Bradycardia, sinus arrest, VF
2. Management
   a. Stop surgery

    b.   Increase depth of anesthesia
    c.   Atropine
    d.   Local anesthetics to eye muscles
    e.   Self-extinguish

Intraocular Gas Expansion
1. D/C N_2O 15 min prior gas injection
2. Avoid N_2O for 5 days after air and 10 days after hexafluoride injection

Echothiophate
1. Also inhibits pseudocholinesterase
2. Prolonged effects of sux and mivacurium

Peri-op Peripheral Nerve Injury

1. Ulnar nerve
    a.   Most common peripheral nerve injury
    b.   More in male
    c.   Proper arm positioning and padding cannot totally prevent
2. Brachial plexus
    a.   Associated with arm abduction more than 90 degree and/or lateral head rotation
3. Sciatic and common peroneal nerve
    a.   Associated with lithotomy position
    b.   Paresthesia without motor deficit
4. Evaluation and treatment
    a.   Physical exam
    b.   Neurology consult
    c.   Sensory neuropathy
      - Usually transient
    d.   Motor neuropathy
      - EMG study
        • Positive 2-3 weeks after the injury
      - Usually recover in weeks to months

Septic Shock

Early Goal (NEJM 2001):
1. CVP 8-12 mmHg (crystalloid and/or colloid if < 8 mmHg)
2. MAP > 65 mmHg (vasopressor if < 65 mmHg)
3. $ScvO_2$ > 70% (transfuse until Hct > 30% if $ScvO_2$ < 70%)

Treatment Updates
1. Hydrocortisone has no benefit (NEJM 2008)
2. Vasopressin is not more beneficial than norepinephrine (NEJM 2008)

3. Conventional insulin therapy (morning blood glucose **151 mg/dl**) is better than intensive insulin therapy (morning blood glucose **112 mg/dl**) (NEJM 2008)
4. Colloid is more likely to cause ARF than LR (NEJM 2008)
5. Protein C is only useful in high APACHE II score pt (NEJM 2005)

Chronic Pain

Chronic Low Back Pain
1. History (www.rad.neuro.com)
    a. Where is the pain?
    b. What kind of pain? Sharp, dull, shooting, or burning pain?
    c. When does the pain occur?
    d. Radiation: Does pain go down to the legs?
    e. Neurological deficit: Any numbness or weakness of the legs? Any urinary or bowel incontinence?
2. Physical examination
    a. Tenderness
    b. Range of motion
    c. Neuro tests: motor and sensory
    d. Specific tests: straight leg raising test, Patrick test
3. Imaging study
    a. Lumbar spine MRI or CT
    b. Lumbar spine X-ray
4. Differential
    a. Disk herniation
    b. Facet joint disease
    c. Sacroiliac joint disease
    d. Spinal stenosis
5. Treatment
    a. Interventional treatment
        - Epidural steroid injection
        - Facet joint injection
        - Sacroiliac joint injection
        - Spinal cord stimulation
    b. Medication
        - Neuropathic medications: neurontin, amitriptyline
        - Central acting muscle relaxant
        - NSAID
        - Narcotics
    c. Surgery
    d. Other
        - Physical therapy
        - Pain psychology
        - Acupuncture

Complex Regional Pain Syndrome (CRPS)

1. Types
    a. Type I (RSD – reflex sympathetic dystrophy): h/o minor injury
    b. Type II (causalgia): h/o major nerve injury
2. Signs and symptoms
    a. Allodynia (painful sensation to non-painful stimuli)
    b. Hyperalgesia (↑ pain sensation to painful stimuli)
    c. Spontaneous pain
    d. Edema
    e. Autonomic dysfunction
    f. Trophic changes
3. Treatment
    a. Intervention
        - Sympathetic block
            • Lumbar sympathetic block for LE
            • Stellate ganglion block for facial and UE
        - Spinal cord stimulation
    b. Medication
        - Neurontin /Lyrica
        - TCA
        - Avoid narcotics

Appendix – ABA Sample Examination

Session 1

CASE:

A 56-year-old, 70 Kg, 5'8" tall man is brought to the operating room for a left upper lobectomy.

HPI: Patient noted the onset of a productive cough 6 weeks ago and an episode of hemoptysis 10 days ago. He was seen by a pulmonary specialist who noted a 2 cm mass in his left upper lobe on chest x-ray. Fiberoptic bronchoscopy revealed irregularity of the left upper lobe bronchus, and biopsy revealed carcinoma. Metastatic workup was negative.

PMH: Uncomplicated myocardial infarction 4 months ago. He notes angina with exercise over past month. A stress test 7 days ago showed minimal ST segment depression at a heart rate of 120 beats per min. without angina. An echocardiogram revealed an ejection fraction of 55%.

Medications include diltiazem and nitroglycerin PRN. He has no allergies.

He smoked 2 packs of cigarettes per day for 25 years until 10 days ago. He drinks an occasional beer.

PHYS EXAM: P 72, BP 140/80, R 20, T 37.1°C. His airway appears normal. Chest auscultation reveals expiratory wheezes over left posterior upper lung field. Cardiac exam is normal. He has no organomegaly or peripheral edema.

X-RAY: 2 cm mass and small infiltrate left upper lobe

EKG: Q waves in II, III, aVf with T wave inversion in same leads.

LABS: Hgb 14.5 gms/dl, normal electrolytes and normal coagulation studies.

He arrives in operating room at 10:00 A.M. with 1" nitropaste, having taken his diltiazem at 7:00 A.M.

QUESTIONS:

Intra-operative Management – 10 Minutes

1. <u>Induction</u>: Would you induce with thiopental? Why/Why not? Propofol? Your choice? Why? The surgeon requests double-lumen tube. You respond? How do you confirm position? Is a right-sided tube appropriate? Why/why not?

2. <u>Anesthetic Selection</u>: Is nitrous oxide-opioid anesthesia appropriate? Why/why not? Your choice? Why? Would halothane be preferable if patient has reactive airway disease? Prefer another inhalation agent in this patient? Why?

3. <u>Intra-operative Hypoxia</u>: After 20 minutes of one-lung ventilation, SpO_2 decreased from 99% to 90%. Your interpretation and response? Rationale for therapeutic choices. What if SpO_2 is 80%?

4. <u>Massive Blood Loss</u>: The surgeon loses control of the pulmonary vein and the patient loses 1200 ml blooding two minutes. Two units of packed cells are available. How to manage? Why? Blood pressure not responding to volume replacement. Your plan? Rationale. Ischemia on ECG. How does it influence your management? Your plan? Why?

Post-operative Care – 15 Minutes

1. <u>Extubation Criteria</u>: How will you decide suitability for extubation? Rationale. How does criteria for this patient differ from ASA-1 cholecystectomy patient? Explain.

2. <u>Post-operative Ventilatory Support</u>: Assume ABG at end of surgery with double-lumen ET tube and bilateral ventilation shows PaO_2 65, $PaCO_2$ 58, pH 7.29 with FIO_2 50% and spontaneous ventilation. Interpret. How will you proceed? Why? If decide to ventilate in ICU will you change ET tube? Why/Why not? Discuss ventilatory settings. Discuss IMV vs. PCV. Discuss PEEP.

3. <u>Pain Management</u>: Would PCA be a good choice? Why/Why not? Is thoracic epidural a better choice? Why/Why not? If epidural in place, what medications would you administer? Why?

4. <u>Myocardial Ischemia</u>: 8 hours after surgery patient complains of anterior chest pain and you note new S-T segment elevation on bedside monitor. How will you proceed? Why? 30 minutes later, his blood pressure is 80/30 and you note tachypnea and diffuse rales. Discuss evaluation and management.

5. <u>Nerve Injury</u>: Following extubation and at time of discharge from ICU, the patient complains of numbness over ulnar distribution of right forearm and hand. What might be the causes? How will you evaluate? Is there any treatment for this? What will you tell patient?

6. <u>Jaundice</u>: 4 days after surgery, the patient's bilirubin is 6.5 mg/dl. Surgeon questions if anesthesia might be the cause. You respond? Discuss further evaluation.

Additional Topics – 10 Minutes

1. <u>Obstetrical Anesthesia - Pre-eclampsia</u>: Urgent C/S for fetal distress is scheduled for 19-year-old parturient who is pre-eclamptic and in active labor. She is receiving MgS04 and intermittent hydralazine. Blood pressure is 150/110. What would be your choice of anesthesia? Why? Discuss advantages/disadvantages of epidural. How would you control blood pressure? Why? What are your goals? Explain.

2. <u>Post-CABG tamponade</u>: A 65-year-old man underwent an uncomplicated CABG 16 hours earlier and was extubated 4 hours ago. In the past hour his BP fell from 110/70 to 70/50 and the CVP rose from 8 to 22 mmHg. What are the possible etiologies? How would you evaluate? Manage? If tamponade is suspected and mediastinal exploration is required, how would you provide anesthesia? Explain.

3. <u>Temperature</u>: A 48-year-old man is undergoing a radical prostatectomy during general anesthesia. Two hours into the operation, his esophageal temperature is 34.5°C. Would you treat? Why/Why not? If so, how? Thirty minutes later it has decreased to 33.5°C. Your management? Surgeon attributes a problem with bleeding to the hypothermia. Agree? Why/Why not? What might be the mechanism? Explain. How will decreased temperature influence your plans for extubation? Describe.

Session 2

CASE:

A 38-year-old, 50 Kg woman is scheduled for excision of an occipital glioma while in the sitting position. You are first to note a late systolic murmur, loudest at left sternal border. She has mild controlled hypertension.

Medications include hydrochlorothiazide for 5 years and dexamethasone for 5 days.

P 74, BP 135/80, R 16, Temp 37°C, Hgb 13 gm/dl, Na 140 mEq/l, K$^+$ 2.9 mEq/l.

QUESTIONS:

Pre-operative Evaluation – 10 minutes
1. Cardiac Status: Neurosurgeon asks what cardiac evaluation is needed. You respond? How does it affect your plan? Do you agree with sitting position? What if no intracardiac defect? Concerns if aortic stenosis is present?
2. ICP: How do you determine if ICP is increased preoperatively? Why important? If evidence for elevation, what steps could you take to reduce? Rationale.
3. Hypokalemia: Are you concerned about K^+ 2.9? Why/Why not? If so, explain. Would you delay surgery until corrected? What would be the endpoint of therapy? Explain. How would you manage K^+ if increase in ICP indicated need for emergency operation?
4. Hypertension: What are the implications of hypertension to anesthetic management? What if blood pressure 180/115? How would you proceed? Explain.

Intra-operative Management – 15 minutes
1. Monitoring: Use PA or multi-orifice CVP catheter? Which? Why? During right IJ cannulation, patient coughs and becomes dyspneic. DDx? Would you obtain a CXR? Why/Why not? Blood pressure declines precipitously. Rx? Rationale.
2. Anesthesia Induction: Special precautions for this patient? Is propofol a good choice? If not, what would you select? Why? Lidocaine helpful? Intravenous or intratracheal? Opioid just as effective? Why/Why not? Is midazolam of any value? Why/Why not?
3. Anesthesia Maintenance: N_2O contraindicated? Why/why not? If so, is "balanced anesthesia" ruled out? Is relaxation needed? Why/Why not? Your management? Rationale.
4. ICP: Surgeon complains that the dura is taut. Your response (Rx)? How much hyperventilation is enough? Deepening anesthesia appropriate? Would you give mannitol? How much? Is there a maximum dose? Why? Is deliberate hypotension beneficial to decrease ICP? Management? How would you accomplish? Why?
5. Hypotension: Sudden blood pressure decrease to 50/35. DDx? Mechanism? How establish Dx air embolism? Presume air embolism has occurred. How would you manage? Why is air embolism risk greater with cranial operation than with other surgical sites if patient is prone? DDx? Tx?
6. Fluid Therapy: What fluid would you use for maintenance? Why? Dextrose content important? Why? How would you differentiate osmotic diuresis from overhydration? How do you determine correct amount of fluid to administer in this situation?

Additional Topics – 10 minutes
1. Pediatric Anesthesia - T - E Fistula: What are the major anesthetic risks for a patient with T-E fistula? Does the type of fistula alter approach? How? A 2.5 Kg newborn from a 34-week gestation presents with an "H" type fistula. Would you

insist on any specific preanesthetic preparations? Which? Why? How would you induce anesthesia? Is a circle system appropriate? Why/Why not? Plans for post-op extubation or continued mechanical ventilation? Rationale for each.

2. <u>Outpatient Regional Anesthesia</u>: A healthy 25-year-old man requests epidural anesthesia for repair of an inguinal hernia as an outpatient. Agree? Why/Why not? If choose epidural, what drugs? Why? Criteria used to discharge patient to home? Suppose an inadvertent dural puncture occurs. What would you do? Would you do a prophylactic blood patch? Why/why not? Would you admit patient to hospital? Why/Why not?

3. <u>Anaphylactic reaction</u>: You are called urgently to radiology where you find a 25-year-old woman undergoing an arteriogram for upper extremity ischemia. She is hypotensive with urticaria, stridor and sternal retraction. What would you do? What is the likely cause? Mechanism of signs and symptoms? Rationale. How proceed if cardiac arrest

Trauma: - Airway - C-spine
           - Transfusion
           - A-Line / Central Line

Allways: low UOP:
           Hx - Fluid Challenge
           - Lasix
           if it doesn't work more fluids
           if not ⇒ Dialysis

VC injury! -
           - Bowel sounds ↑ENT consult
           - Indirect laryngoscopy Bedside

Dermatome Reproductive Organs or else more.
              ~~T6~~ ~~T10~~ T-6